A Few Words from Active Moms

Hello Readers,

Prior to working with Ashley, I was a runner and that was it—I didn't know where to even start when it came to strength training. Her Core, Function, and Fitness Method not only taught me how to train with proper techniques, emphasizing the importance of breathing, it was also the inspiration for my mama mantra of, "strong, not skinny." She built this fierce community of active moms meeting early in the morning with the best play lists ever—our conversations were just as important as our workouts—and she made it fun. Ashley's method gave me strength and confidence to function every day in city life, from taking the stroller on the subway to carrying groceries and that heavy infant car seat across town. I never realized how much getting stronger would help me emotionally deal with so many phases of motherhood, marriage, and hormonal rollercoasters during pregnancy and beyond.

    I was in the best shape of my life while training with Ashley from postpartum with my first baby through a pandemic pregnancy and boom—life changed in an instant when I was diagnosed with stage 3 breast cancer. Ashley and her approach to exercise supported me every step of the way. I'm so proud to call Ashley my trainer, coach, and dear friend!

—**Shannon Gottesman**, mom of two

Dear Readers,

I never thought I'd be able to do a sit-up again after having kids, but Ashley's Core, Function, and Fitness method helped me rebuild my core and confidence. The Active Mom community gave me strength and grounded me—not just physically, but mentally and emotionally—especially during a harder second pregnancy and several job and life changes. My kids tried joining my workouts and quickly dropped out because they were too hard! I started training with Ashley so I could pick up my kids and keep up with them. Now, after several years postpartum, I continue applying Core, Function, and Fitness for me. I am a woman, mom, wife, daughter, professional, and so much more—and I am strong.

—**Susan Hines**, mom of two

Active Mom

Your Guide to Feeling Strong and Confident in Pregnancy, Postpartum, and Beyond

Ashley Reid

BLOOMSBURY ACADEMIC
NEW YORK • LONDON • OXFORD • NEW DELHI • SYDNEY

BLOOMSBURY ACADEMIC

Bloomsbury Publishing Inc, 1359 Broadway, 12th Floor, New York, NY 10018, USA
Bloomsbury Publishing Plc, 50 Bedford Square, London, WC1B 3DP, UK
Bloomsbury Publishing Ireland, 29 Earlsfort Terrace, Dublin 2, D02 AY28, Ireland

BLOOMSBURY, BLOOMSBURY ACADEMIC and the Diana logo are trademarks of
Bloomsbury Publishing Plc

First published in the United States of America 2026

Copyright © Ashley Reid, 2026

Cover design: Jen Huppert
Cover images: © istock/manonallard, © istock/Courtney Hale,
© istock/Prostock-Studio, © istock/RyanJLane

All rights reserved. No part of this publication may be: i) reproduced or transmitted in any form, electronic or mechanical, including photocopying, recording or by means of any information storage or retrieval system without prior permission in writing from the publishers; or ii) used or reproduced in any way for the training, development or operation of artificial intelligence (AI) technologies, including generative AI technologies. The rights holders expressly reserve this publication from the text and data mining exception as per Article 4(3) of the Digital Single Market Directive (EU) 2019/790.

Bloomsbury Publishing Inc does not have any control over, or responsibility for, any third-party websites referred to or in this book. All internet addresses given in this book were correct at the time of going to press. The author and publisher regret any inconvenience caused if addresses have changed or sites have ceased to exist, but can accept no responsibility for any such changes.

A catalog record for this book is available from the Library of Congress.

ISBN: HB: 979-8-8818-0809-9
ePDF: 979-8-2163-7474-9
eBook: 979-8-8818-0810-5

Typeset by Deanta Global Publishing Services, Chennai, India
Printed and bound in the United States of America

For product safety related questions contact productsafety@bloomsbury.com.

To find out more about our authors and books visit www.bloomsbury.com and sign up for our newsletters.

Contents

Foreword by Linda E. May vii
Acknowledgments ix
Author's Note xi

Introduction 1

Part I

1 What Does It Mean to Be an Active Mom? 13
2 An Approach to Exercise That Supports Motherhood 19
3 Figuring Out What You Need 29

Part II

4 Your Core from the Inside Out 47
5 It's Not Just You and You Don't Have to Live with It 59
6 Core Training for Moms 89

Part III

7   Master These (Mom) Movements 115
8   Isolated Muscle Training for Strength and Mobility 135
9   When to Push, Pause, or Pivot 151

Part IV

10   What about Cardio? 187
11   Putting It All Together 203

Appendix A: My Letters to You 231
Appendix B: Additional Resources 240
Notes 243
Bibliography 252
Index 258
About the Author 263

Foreword

Linda E. May, PhD, MS, FAHA

*Dr. **Linda May**, associate professor in the Kinesiology Department of Health and Human Performance at East Carolina University, teaches exercise physiology students and is adjunct faculty in obstetrics and gynecology for the Brody School of Medicine. Ashley Reid and Dr. May met as members of the American College of Sports Medicine Pregnancy and Postpartum Special Interest Group, and Ashley has enjoyed sharing her practical maternal exercise findings with Linda's students.*

Numerous advances have been made in the field of exercise during pregnancy and the postpartum period since the 1970s. Although scientific knowledge has increased, this information has not always been translated back to pregnant women or their healthcare providers. Therefore, healthcare providers and pregnant women need to know what they can and should be doing to stay active during and after their pregnancy.

This book will provide a foundation and framework to know what can and should be done to stay active during your pregnancy and after your baby is born. You will start by understanding what it means to be active and what the current recommendations are for maternal exercise. You will also learn about your body core and how to train this effectively for improved pregnancy outcomes and overall health before and after your pregnancy. Importantly, exercise is not "one-size-fits-all," and you will learn what is right for you, your body, and this pregnancy. This book will help you start your path to being happier and healthier during and after your pregnancy to be an Active Mom!

Acknowledgments

When I made it my mission to provide moms with the support they deserve, I also set out to gain as much experience and knowledge as possible, and to make that information accessible to moms everywhere. I'm incredibly grateful to have had the opportunity to do so, and getting to this point took the support and trust of many.

This may seem obvious once you read the introduction, but the first person I want to thank is my daughter, Hayden. In addition to directly inspiring my work with moms and moms-to-be, she has been my most authentic supporter, even as a young child. From sitting on stacks of tile while I built out my studio, to early Saturday mornings watching me lead prenatal and postpartum groups, to bringing me snacks while I wrote this book and asking how many chapters I finished that day when I picked her up from school, she has been part of this mission every step of the way. I'm so grateful to her.

And to my mom, thank you for giving me the confidence to pursue new endeavors and the encouragement to never shy away from them. Who would have guessed that the stories you encouraged me to write as a kid would turn into something so meaningful? I love you, Mom.

To the maternal health researchers, especially Linda E. May, PhD, MS, FAHA, thank you for not only advancing the field of maternal exercise but also for mentoring the next generation of researchers who are continuing to push boundaries. And to Margie Davenport, PhD, your body of work is both impressive and impactful. You are a true advocate, and I've been honored to take your research and translate it into real-world support for moms. Your work provides direction, reduces fear, and empowers action—thank you.

To Philly's incredible prenatal and postpartum healthcare professionals, especially the pelvic floor physical therapists, your collaboration has shaped my approach in meaningful ways. Your dedication, expertise, and compassion are making a real impact. I've been fortunate to team up with outstanding providers at Axia Women's Health, Bridge, Ivy Rehab for Women's Health, Restore Physical Therapy and Pelvic Health, Pelvio Physical Therapy, Excel Physical Therapy, Atlantic Physical Therapy, Good Shepherd Penn Partners, Jefferson Health, and Penn Medicine. Thank you.

To the team who brought this book to life, Katharine Sands with Sarah Jane Freymann Literary Agency, you believed in this project from the moment I shared the idea and championed it with care. I'm so grateful you saw its value and worked to find the right home. Christen Karniski, Joanna Wattenberg, and the entire team at Bloomsbury, thank you for truly understanding the message behind this book and allowing me to tell it in my own voice. It's been a pleasure working with you.

To all the Active Moms I've had the privilege of supporting, whether in person or virtually, individually or in groups, at your house or in my studio, for six weeks or six years, you've each played an essential role in this movement and the growth of the Active Mom Fitness community. You're the reason I kept showing up, and you've inspired me more than you know.

And to the reader, thank you for allowing me to be a part of your motherhood journey, and welcome to the Active Mom Fitness Community.

Author's Note

This book is designed to inform and empower, but it is not a substitute for individualized medical advice. Every mother's body, pregnancy, and postpartum recovery is unique.

The movement strategies and exercise practices shared here are intended to help you make informed, personal decisions about your health and fitness. For most women, physical activity is safe, beneficial, and should not be feared.

If you have medical concerns, develop new symptoms, or are unsure whether you have a health condition that may affect your ability to exercise, consult with your healthcare provider for guidance.

Introduction

Whether you're still crafting your pregnancy announcement, reading this during newborn naps, or maybe you've been trying to juggle your kids and fitness for years, I want to start by telling you that you should be proud of yourself for starting this book. You're choosing to prioritize your health, wellness, and fitness for the good of you and your family, and that's a significant undertaking. Your fitness and motherhood journey will go through stages and phases, and this book is a resource that I hope you can refer back to whenever you need guidance. Every time you pick up this book, remind yourself that you have the right to understand and feel empowered in your body. When the mom guilt creeps in, don't forget that taking care of yourself isn't a luxury, it's essential. As you reread the chapters most applicable to you, know that there are hundreds of moms experiencing similar challenges and that no matter where you are in your motherhood or fitness journey, you now belong to an inspiring community of Active Moms.

Hello. My name is Ashley Reid, and I'm an Exercise Physiologist, Pre/Postnatal Wellness Practitioner, and mother of one. I am also the founder of Active Mom Fitness®, which began as a private and small group strength training studio for moms and moms-to-be and grew to a brand providing education and empowerment to moms and those who support moms. If we were speaking in person, you could think of these first few pages as just the beginning of our ongoing conversation. In this introduction, I'll share just a little bit about me personally and professionally, because after all, you are entrusting me to support you during a significant time in your life. I'll also share why I wrote the book, who I wrote it for, and how you can use the Active Mom Guide to be strong, fit, and confident in pregnancy, postpartum, and beyond. Let's get started!

Why I Wrote This Book

In short, I wrote this book because I developed an approach to exercise that works, and I want it to be accessible to all moms. You deserve the knowledge and tools to understand your body so that you can make informed decisions about your fitness throughout every stage of motherhood. The physical and emotional demands of motherhood change over time. From the anatomical shifts during pregnancy to postpartum recovery, extending into the physical and emotional demands of caring for your child(ren), moms are in constant transition, and your approach to fitness should reflect that. Exercise can be your most powerful tool to help you adapt and thrive at every stage. My background is in strength and conditioning, and similar to how an athlete's training cycle is designed to prevent injury, develop specific skills, and improve overall fitness, a mom's fitness routine should take that same approach. Exercise selection should prevent injuries caused by repetitive movements like lifting your child off the floor. Fitness programs should take into account the anatomical changes of pregnancy and sleep deprivation. We can, and should, train for the sport of motherhood. I wrote this guide to address your evolving needs.

Who This Guide Is For

First, let's make sure we're on the same page when we talk about the terms prenatal and postpartum. Generally, everyone agrees that prenatal refers to the time you are pregnant. Although this is true, for this book, if you are someone not yet pregnant or trying to conceive, some of the prenatal exercise guidance is relevant to you as well. For example, prenatal fitness strategies like training your pelvic floor muscles or mastering the major movement patterns are beneficial to prepare your body for pregnancy. This guide will provide you with plenty of support if you're reading this before becoming pregnant.

When it comes to postpartum, there is a little less consensus on the definition. The duration of the postpartum period is somewhat vague, and it can range from weeks to months after giving birth. Commonly, people use the term "fourth trimester" to describe the three months post-childbirth. *Webster's Dictionary*[1] defines postpartum as "occurring in or being the period following childbirth." In the context of fitness, postpartum exercise needs can extend beyond what is typically considered postpartum.

In this book, if I provide "postpartum" guidance, that information is relevant to anyone taking their first steps toward fitness after having a baby. For some moms, that might be six weeks after giving birth, and for others, one to two years. For example, if you are in your fourth trimester, my approach would be to focus on deep core activation. I would use a similar approach if you had given birth two years ago but had not yet dedicated time to strengthening the deep core muscles. So, if you're beyond the initial period after birth, understand that you should not define your needs based on time.

If you value guidance rooted in science but still crave simple, practical advice, this book is for you. If you want recommendations from someone who not only understands exercise but also knows firsthand how fatigue and fear can become barriers, then this book is for you. If you're wondering if this book will benefit you, the short answer is yes, I wrote this book for you.

A Heartfelt Thank You

In case it isn't clear yet, I want to welcome you to your Active Mom journey! Together, let's acknowledge that this book wouldn't be possible without the trust that so many moms like you put into me. I spent the first nine years of my daughter's life building a fitness space designed for (not modified for) moms. I had the privilege of coaching and learning from: moms with chronic pain, CrossFit enthusiasts, cancer survivors, stay-at-home moms, moms who've experienced pregnancy loss, business owners, former college athletes, twin moms, moms in uniform, those new to exercise, those battling injuries and surgeries, moms over forty, moms who are marathoners, women going through fertility treatments, and many mothers who trained with me through multiple pregnancy and postpartum periods. These moms counted on me to translate exercise science into practice, affirmed that I could be a mom and entrepreneur, and showed me that what I was doing in the fitness space was needed and appreciated. You'll even hear about some of them in this guide (using pseudonyms). So, as you embark on your motherhood fitness journey, keep in mind that there is another mom like you out there who has let me guide them to strength and confidence, and that they're rooting for you!

My Story

I've always had an interest and appreciation for what the human body can do. I grew up playing sports and was decent enough to enjoy them but didn't excel beyond the high school level. I sprained my ankle several times playing softball and was no stranger to shin splints during track season. In college, I studied exercise science/kinesiology with a concentration in sports medicine and often used myself and my friends as subjects to trial what I was learning. As part of the degree, I was required to take physical activity credits, and my weight training class enlightened me about the power of strength and conditioning in injury prevention (since that class and consistently strength training, I have never experienced shin splints again). After graduation, I became credentialed as a National Strength and Conditioning Association Certified Strength and Conditioning Specialist and Certified Exercise Physiologist by the American College of Sports Medicine. Both are the gold-standard certifications in the fitness industry.

If I were to sum up my career history from corporate wellness to health and physical education, to obesity prevention research projects, to inclusive fitness, I'd say the commonality of all my roles was empowering people through exercise. Through coaching, training, and education, I've helped people ages five to eighty-five prevent injury, increase confidence, lose weight, improve performance, relieve stress, reduce disease risk, and enhance their quality of life. However, it wasn't until I became pregnant with my daughter that I shifted my focus to moms.

During pregnancy, I experienced firsthand the lack of exercise resources and education for moms. Not only is there a shortage of studies specifically on women and exercise, but studies during pregnancy and postpartum are even more scarce. When I became pregnant, I was committed to continuing to workout, but I didn't anticipate the fear and uncertainty around whether the intensity or types of exercise I was doing could negatively impact my pregnancy. I realized that even with the top certifications, education, and professional experience, I was not prepared for prenatal exercise.

There weren't any prenatal fitness classes beyond yoga accessible to me, and I wasn't able to get detailed advice from my doctor. It was clear that even though our OB/Gyns know the value of exercise, and many are keen to recommend it to their patients, they are not trained to provide us with specifics. In all the continuing education and professional coursework that I've done as a fitness professional, there'd only been a handful of opportunities to learn about what exercise should look like during and after pregnancy. The void in the maternal exercise space was evident.

Let's now fast forward to my postpartum experience, where I felt equally unprepared. Everybody's labor and delivery unfold differently, but whether you had a short vaginal delivery or a planned C-section, all moms require healing and a gradual return to physical activity. Once again, I felt unequipped. I was unaware of the type and how much movement I should be doing. To make the situation more challenging, I was recovering from a traumatic C-section after thirty-six hours of labor, so, ideally, I would have received rehabilitative exercise suggestions just as you'd expect after other major surgeries.

Instead of using exercise as a tool to rebuild, I, like many others, just waited until my postpartum appointment and got the go-ahead for exercise and sex, taking it as a green light to do both. Well, let's just say that neither went so well. I chose to follow a twelve-week strength training program designed by a trusted fitness professional I'd admired for years. It wasn't designed specifically for moms, and after struggling through the first workout, I cried. Despite exercising for thirty-nine weeks of pregnancy, the workout felt extremely difficult. In addition, sex was painful. I was incredibly frustrated, thinking I could return to these activities, yet having to accept that my body wasn't ready. So here I was again with another aha moment. I realized that if someone with my background in exercise and access to good healthcare didn't know what type of exercise program would be beneficial or where to turn for the painful sex, then other moms probably felt the same. Thankfully, I was motivated to figure it out.

I can't recall how I found my way to pelvic floor physical therapy, but I'm grateful that I did. At that time, it wasn't as widely known as it is now, and it wasn't seen as a normal part of postpartum care. I won't tell you that it was easy to stay consistent with appointments or the at-home exercises, but it was worth it, and I'm a huge advocate that all moms should be provided with a pelvic floor physical therapy evaluation. But that's not the only point I'm trying to make here. For me, not only was it effective, allowing me a full recovery, but it was also educational. My physical therapist was open to all my questions, and we communicated about what was working and what wasn't. I began to further my learning and increase my understanding of the core and pelvic floor muscles. I ended up taking what I gained from her and applying it to the principles of strength and conditioning to create an exercise plan that finally worked for me. From there, I hosted focus groups with other moms and eventually started leading prenatal and postpartum group training (that even my pelvic floor PT began attending!). I knew I needed to help other moms navigate exercise during and after pregnancy so that they didn't have to feel what I felt. I declared it my mission to help moms and moms-to-be feel strong and confident through all stages of motherhood.

It took a few years of education and practical experience, but I'm proud to say that I developed an approach to mom fitness that has resulted in moms staying active through thirty-nine to forty weeks of pregnancy and returning to fitness safely after having a baby (most feeling stronger than ever before). For those of you new to exercise, if your doctor has said it's safe for you to be physically active, motherhood is a great time to begin. For fitness enthusiasts, rest assured, you can find a way to keep exercising through all stages of motherhood if you follow the right approach.

An exercise program designed specifically for a mom's body benefits your mental and physical health, not just during pregnancy and the fourth trimester but for a lifetime. As my daughter has gotten older, I've been able to (1) meet the physical demands of the toddler years, moving pain free, (2) have the energy and ability to be active with her, even as a busy mom and entrepreneur, and (3) set a healthy example that will benefit her for her lifetime. Being an Active Mom is going to let me keep making memories with her for years to come, and I want the same for you!

Book Structure

Although we all have similar needs and there are common obstacles all of us moms face, fitness is not one-size-fits-all. This guide is meant to educate and empower you so that you can personalize a fitness journey to meet your needs, goals, and stage of motherhood. I want to support and guide you as best I can through the next eleven chapters.

Each chapter will begin with a couple of key insights. This makes it easy to return to the guide and determine which sections to reread. I will cite studies and established guidelines to support my suggestions that have come from practical experience working with moms. I've gotten to know maternal health researchers doing extraordinary work to push the field forward, and I want to do my part to disseminate this information to you. You'll notice that at times I "infer" from research, meaning that while a study's successful outcomes may not have specifically included moms, the findings have been proven in other populations. Based on those results and my experience, it's reasonable to expect similar benefits for moms. I may also infer when offering guidance based on prenatal or postpartum studies that had limitations, such as a small sample size. If you feel empowered to learn more, please explore my references or seek affirmation on the information in this book from physical therapists, fitness professionals, doctors, or other healthcare professionals. Lastly, each chapter will end with suggested next steps to help you put what you've learned into practice.

I'll begin the book by introducing you to the Core, Function, and Fitness® method, which is the framework I've used with moms in the Active Mom Fitness community. I coach you through the mental shift that needs to happen during each stage of motherhood and provide you with a self-assessment so that you can read the book with a personal lens.

In Part II, we take a deep dive into the core. Not only is proper core training crucial for moms, but in my opinion, it is the key to enhancing fitness for everyone. Although it may feel like you'll never get rid of back pain during pregnancy, or that your abs are mushy postpartum, the best part of learning how to train your core correctly is that with the right progression, you have the opportunity to be stronger than you were before pregnancy. In the core chapters, you'll learn how common conditions like incontinence and diastasis recti don't have to hinder physical activity. You'll end these chapters knowing exactly where to start with your core training and how to determine if an exercise is safe and effective for you.

Part III is a section that I hope you continue to refer to as your fitness ability and stage of motherhood change. What I love most about these chapters is that I'm not going to give you a prescriptive workout routine, but rather I'll teach you how to progress and regress your workouts as your time, energy, fitness ability, and body change. Whether you're selecting your exercises, following a workout on an app, or attending group fitness classes, you'll have the ability to determine if the workouts you're doing will give you the results you're seeking. Say goodbye to random modifications, selecting workouts haphazardly, and relying on AI "best exercise" lists.

In Part IV, I explain the last piece of the Core, Function, and Fitness method. It's where everything comes together, and any lingering questions are answered. I will give you the template that personal trainers use to design programs for their clients so that when you're done reading, you'll have a clear, personalized plan of action. Additionally, you'll select strategies and tips that will help you succeed.

I wrote the last section of the letters because although I would love to speak to each of you individually about your needs and goals, I can't. In place of conversation, I wrote letters to connect with and encourage you. As I mentioned, I've been privileged to work with moms from diverse backgrounds and experiences, and as I welcome you to the Active Mom Community, I want to pass on what I've learned from them. If you find a letter that resonates with you, know that it's sincere and that I hope it inspires you to take the next step, whatever that might be.

So, without further ado, I'm grateful for this opportunity to support you. Let's move on to Part I!

Part I

Part 1

1

What Does It Mean to Be an Active Mom?

Key Insights from This Chapter

1. Being an Active Mom is about using exercise as a tool to feel strong and confident in every stage of motherhood.
2. Your fitness goals will shift during pregnancy and postpartum. Instead of focusing on prepregnancy benchmarks, developing new goals will lead to fitness success and sustainability.
3. Your exercise routine should be personal. What worked for someone else may not work for you.

Let's start with a simple activity: I'd like you to close your eyes for ten seconds and think about what you see when you hear "fit mom." What does she look like? What is she doing? How does she interact with her kids? Now, take another ten seconds to visualize an "Active Mom." What does she look like? What is she doing? How does she interact with her kids?

When I founded Active Mom Fitness, I was very intentional about my word choices and chose a name that truly aligned with my mission. The image that comes to *my* mind when I hear "fit mom" or use the term "fit pregnancy" is too specific and is only relatable to some. However, I associate "active" as an inclusive term to describe a mom who is empowered, healthy, and confident in movement. When I think of an "Active Mom," I see someone who enjoys physical activity throughout pregnancy. I see a mom who goes on outdoor walks with her newborn to boost her mood. My vision is of a mother organizing weekend family activities like hiking or biking. I envision a mother who fits in mini workouts during toddler nap time or chooses to walk instead of drive to work. An Active Mom moves through her day without pain and has the energy to play with her child even after a long day of work. An Active Mom adapts her exercise routine as she goes through various stages of motherhood, setting an example for her family. Active Moms are the grandmothers still chasing their grandkids on the playground and being full participants on family trips. Sure, like a "fit mom," an Active Mom may also prioritize a specific aesthetic or physique, might be an avid gymgoer, and set fitness goals like running marathons, but her "why" encompasses so much more than that.

The concept is simple: To be an Active Mom, you must use exercise as your most powerful tool. Active Moms challenge their bodies in a way that is effective and beneficial. They feel confident and strong in their changing bodies. Active Moms value exercise and activity and are committed to making it a lifestyle. Are you ready to join the Active Mom community?

The Mental Shift

The first step in your Active Mom journey is mental. If we're being honest with ourselves, becoming a mom comes with physical *and* emotional changes, so the fitness goals we had before pregnancy should not be the same benchmarks we use during or after. This can be difficult for someone who has been active their entire life and has previously only set goals based on performance, weight loss, or physique. It can be a real identity shift. The same goes for someone without much exercise experience. You may mentally feel the pressure to stay active because you know it's good for you and the baby, but if the gym has never been your happy place, it can be challenging to find the confidence and motivation to begin a program. However, the sooner that you can acknowledge that exercise during the first few years of motherhood will play a different role than it does at other points in your life, the more realistic and manageable your goals will be and the more effective your exercise program will be.

If you're a fitness fanatic and this sounds unsettling to you, don't worry, I'm not saying exercise can't be a priority or that you can't enjoy workouts that push your limits. It's quite the opposite. I'm just saying that as you go through the physical and emotional changes of motherhood, shifting your "why" and adapting your exercise plan will ensure your success.

So now it's time to ask yourself, how can exercise be your tool? What goals make the most sense for you? How will your current routine shift to meet those goals? If you're beyond childbirth, ask yourself if your fitness goals are realistic. Have they changed from your prepregnancy or pregnancy activity goals?

Common Prenatal Exercise Goals

- "I want to prepare for labor."
- "I want to better my chances for a smooth postpartum recovery."
- "I don't want to gain too much weight."

- "I want to prevent gestational diabetes."
- "I want to feel in control of my body."
- "I need to relieve stress."
- "I want my core to stay strong and protect my abs from separation."
- "I want to have a healthy pregnancy and healthy baby."

Common Postpartum Exercise Goals

- "I just want to feel like myself again."
- "I want more energy."
- "My abs feel mushy, and I want to connect with them again."
- "I need to strengthen my pelvic floor."
- "I want to be able to wear my baby without back pain."
- "I want to figure out how to make time for a consistent exercise routine."
- "I need to fix my posture after breastfeeding."

Make It Personal

Hopefully, by now, you are feeling motivated to be an Active Mom and make the mental shift to use exercise as your ally. So, the last point I'll make is that your program has to be personal. As moms, we LOVE to give advice and suggestions to other moms, with good intentions, of course. However, what worked for your best friend or what your mom recommends is not tailored to your specific needs. So lean on your mom tribe for support and inspiration, but when it comes to the details of your fitness plan, ensure your exercise program aligns with your personal goals.

No need to answer these questions now, but let's start to reframe our perspective and begin looking at exercise from a personal lens. What are your physical weaknesses? What type of activity do you already do during the day? What pregnancy complications do/did you have? What type of birth complications did you have? What's your energy like? Do you have childcare? What exercise experience do you have? Do you have diastasis recti or pelvic floor dysfunction? Do you have more time for exercise now that your kids are older?

All these factors will determine when, what, and how much exercise you do. Your time and energy as a mom are precious, and if you're going to put effort into exercising it better be effective and work for *you*. If that feels overwhelming, have no fear . . . this book is going to guide you through each step. Let's keep going!

Take Action

Choose one of the prompts below and write your response on a sticky note. Place the sticky note where you'll see it every day.

1. Define what "Active Mom" means to you. Write down three words or phrases that capture the image that came to mind when you visualized your version of an Active Mom.
2. List three benefits of exercise you value right now.

2

An Approach to Exercise That Supports Motherhood

Key Insights from This Chapter

1. The gap between fitness and maternal healthcare means many moms don't receive the exercise guidance they need, leading to uncertainty and inactivity.
2. Strength training is an essential form of exercise for moms at all stages of motherhood.
3. Your fitness approach should be flexible and evolve with your needs. The Core, Function and Fitness® (CFF) method helps you prioritize what matters most at each stage of motherhood.

You're reading this book because you care about staying active and strong throughout motherhood, but let's be honest, exercise guidelines are broad and general, so even though you value exercise, you may not understand what these recommendations look like in real life. What does resistance training look like during pregnancy? How do you achieve the amount of exercise recommended by your doctor?

How do you stay consistent with pelvic floor exercise? If you don't feel confident in your answers to those questions, you are not alone, and that's why this book is so important.

In a study of 1,510 pregnant women, 60 percent of them reported not being physically active during pregnancy, and one of the main reasons mentioned in that study is that they didn't have enough information and knowledge from their doctors to be physically active.[1] Your doctor's top priority is making sure the baby is developing as it should and the mom remains healthy, but their exercise training is often limited or nonexistent.[2] I didn't need this research to know that exercise is not a core piece of medical training. Of all professions, the medical field was one of the top industries represented among my clients. I coached cardiologists, sports medicine doctors, emergency medicine specialists, and oncologists. I attribute this to those moms understanding the changes the body goes through, and the importance of physical activity, but also acknowledging that they are not equipped with the knowledge to formulate a safe and effective prenatal or postpartum exercise plan. They recognized the importance of selecting a program they can remain consistent with and appreciated the need to develop strategies to hold themselves accountable. So again, I'm not knocking the medical profession but rather validating your inaction, inconsistency, fear, and uncertainty. If you've been told by your physician that it is safe for you to exercise during or after pregnancy, or that exercise is the solution to better physical or mental health, but you don't know what your next steps should be, know that many moms feel that way. By the time you finish this book, you'll have the knowledge and confidence to take your next step forward with clarity and direction.

Some of you may be fortunate enough to have found an exercise professional who specializes in pre- and postnatal fitness (and not just someone who knows exercise and happens to have had a baby).

If that's the case, you have a great advantage because, as I already alluded to, there is a gap between fitness and maternal healthcare and between research and practice. The anatomical and physiological changes a mom's body goes through are significant, and I hope we reach a point where every professional working in maternal health, fitness, or wellness is a true specialist, fully equipped to understand those changes and provide the care moms deserve. Until we reach that point, you must be an advocate for yourself.

To be an advocate for your health and fitness, you need to feel empowered. You also need to be knowledgeable so that you can create, choose, or participate in exercise programs that address not just the changes your body goes through but also those that factor in family and life demands. To help you with this, I want to share with you what I believe to be the top ten benefits of strength training . . . there are more than this list. Then, after I convert you into a strength training enthusiast, I will give you the approach to prenatal, postpartum, and motherhood fitness so that even if you're not working with a specialist, you'll know how to begin to put exercise guidelines into practice.

Why Strength Training?

I believe that strength training is the most important type of exercise for moms. Not only have I seen the benefits firsthand, but they're also backed by research, and, honestly, they just make sense. At the time of writing this guide, the World Health Organization recommends that adults do "muscle-strengthening activities at moderate or greater intensity that involve all major muscle groups on 2 or more days a week." Additionally, it recommends that pregnant and postpartum people without contraindications "incorporate a variety of aerobic and muscle-strengthening activities."[3]

Here are ten reasons why you should commit to strength training during the natal period and beyond:

1. Strength training can help reduce pregnancy-related low back pain. Your body goes through significant anatomical changes during pregnancy, including an increased curve in your lower back, which can lead to discomfort or pain. Strengthening your muscles, especially in your legs and glutes,[4] plays a key role in supporting your spine and reducing the common aches and pains that many moms experience during pregnancy.

2. Strength training helps you meet the physical demands of caring for a child. Caring for a child involves repetitive lifting, bending, and carrying throughout the day, for years. By improving your strength, you'll make these tasks easier and enhance your overall quality of life.

3. Strength training plays a role in supporting healthy weight management. During pregnancy, resistance training can help ward off excessive gestational weight gain.[5] For moms postpartum and beyond, resistance training helps promote fat loss while preserving lean muscle mass. This means that instead of losing muscle along with fat, your body maintains more of its strength and shape as you lose weight. Think of strength training as a long-term strategy for weight control and body composition.[6]

4. Resistance training naturally engages and strengthens your pelvic floor muscles through core activation. Stabilizing during strength exercises increases intra-abdominal pressure (which you'll learn more about in Chapters 4 and 5), triggering a coordinated response from your core. Studies show that in healthy women, pelvic floor muscles contract alongside

abdominal muscles, meaning your strength workouts support your pelvic health.[7]

5. Strength training can help you restore a sense of control over your body. It isn't uncommon for me to hear from moms and moms-to-be that they don't "feel" their muscles firing. Whether this is due to the mind-body connection being disrupted or because of physical changes, beginning a strength training program helps them "feel" the right muscles. I always tell people that an exercise isn't mastered until you can "feel" the right muscles activating at the right time. Studies show that strength training helps build your neuromuscular pathways and that, rather than just going through the motions without thought, you can increase the ability to develop strength and definition by focusing on the working muscle.[8]

6. Building strength supports your posture and balance as your body changes during pregnancy. As your belly and breasts grow, your center of gravity shifts, placing more demand on muscles that didn't have to work as hard before.[9] Strength training helps improve stability and coordination, making it easier to move confidently and stay steady.

7. Strength training is a physical activity with a long list of health benefits. As moms, we all want to enjoy as much time as possible with our children. We want to be able not just to be there but also to be present and make memories. To do that, we need to value our health. Performing resistance training two to three days per week can prevent, manage, and treat arthritis, cancers, cardiovascular diseases, depression, diabetes, high blood pressure, insomnia, osteoporosis, and other conditions.[10]

8. Resistance training is a great low-impact addition to your routine if you're avoiding activities like running or jumping. Whether

you're pregnant and running causes incontinence, breastfeeding and jumping feel uncomfortable, or approaching menopause and no longer enjoy high-impact workouts like you used to, strength training benefits your bones without the impact.

9. Strength training positively impacts your immune system, which is especially important during pregnancy, while healing postpartum, and for fighting off the germs your little ones bring home from school. While research hasn't focused specifically on moms, studies show that even a single workout can enhance immune cell activity. With consistent strength training over several weeks, you'll experience long-lasting improvements in immunity and reduced inflammation.[11]

10. Lastly, strength training is highly adaptable, with endless variations in resistance, tempo, and equipment. This means you can adjust your routine, progressing or scaling back as needed to match your stage of motherhood. If you're not dealing with injuries or complications, strength training is one of the few forms of exercise you'll rarely need to pause completely . . . hello, consistency! As a mom, it can be tough to squeeze in a run without childcare, or attending your favorite 7 p.m. yoga class might feel less appealing if it means missing your baby's bedtime. Strength training, on the other hand, can be done at home with minimal equipment, making it an ideal way for moms to stay active and consistent.

Have I convinced you yet? I sure hope so because now I will introduce you to a method that I've named and trademarked "Core, Function and Fitness" (CFF). By following the CFF framework, you'll determine your starting point and learn how to progress your routine, so you continue to get results. This method will help you identify your fitness priorities and select exercises based on your individual needs. You can apply this approach to gym workouts, home workouts, or programs on an app, or provided by AI.

CFF can be visualized as three components in a pie chart, with the percentage of each changing based on your need and stage of motherhood. It can also be understood as a progression, beginning with one component and moving on to the next. I often explain it as a pyramid with the base being the foundational component of your exercise program.

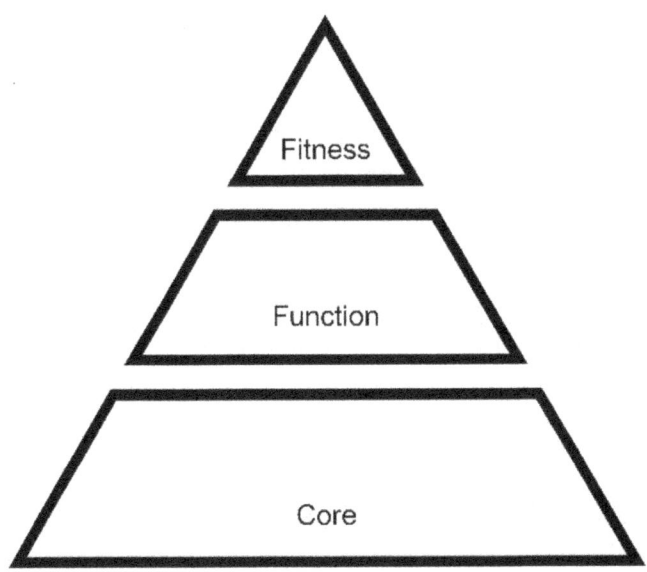

The CFF framework: Core, Function and Fitness. This model represents the foundational approach to training through motherhood, beginning with core, progressing to function, and then building toward fitness goals. Created by author on Canva; © Ashley Reid.

Core

When I refer to your "core," I'm talking about the 360-degree cylinder that runs from your diaphragm to your pelvic floor, including both your abdominal and back muscles. This part of CFF focuses on choosing exercises or following a program that improves both the strength and function of your core muscles. For example, not only do your abdominal muscles need to be strong, but they should also coordinate with your breath for optimal function. Your core strength and function impact everything from daily tasks to workouts, which is why "core" is the base of the pyramid, the first step in the linear progression, or initially the largest portion of your pie chart.

Function

Moving to the "function" piece of my approach assumes that you have foundational core strength and function. This component prioritizes functional training, so you can meet the physical demands of your life. These demands might include occupational activity, like being a mail carrier or home health aide. For others, the discomfort that comes from sitting in front of a computer all day may need to be addressed through functional training. If we're looking specifically at motherhood tasks, functional training during pregnancy includes exercises that help you adapt to the changes your body is experiencing. If you've had a baby, your functional needs will continue to change based on the age of your child, and incorporating an exercise program that helps you lift, carry, and chase your child is what I'd consider training for function.

"Function" is the second step in the CFF model because you should feel good moving through your daily life with limited discomfort before moving to typical fitness goals. As an example, by the time my daughter was about eleven months old, I was consistently doing a spin class once per week among other formats of exercise, and I was moving toward more vigorous fitness goals. This was until I suffered a back injury during a car accident. As a result of the injury, I had a hard time lifting my daughter without pain and moved more slowly doing daily tasks. So, although at the time of the accident I was ready and preparing to advance to the third component at the top of the pyramid, due to the injury, I had to reprioritize. I chose to return to the foundational level and made "core" the focus of my workouts again. I knew that some positions on the spin bike would do no favors to my back, so I replaced that workout with core exercises and mobility work. By returning to the first component of the framework, I was able to continue with exercise and heal from the injury.

Fitness

In CFF, "fitness" is the component that usually comes to mind when people think of exercise. When I speak of "fitness" as part of the Core, Function and Fitness method, it signifies the advancement or progression to goals like increased muscle definition, weight loss, and enhanced sports performance. Training in this category might consist of advanced lifting routines, longer or more frequent cardio sessions, training for a sport or race, and following a more specific diet. Many moms fail at fitness because they go into fitness with the mentality that this is the first step, when really, I've seen moms have more success achieving these goals after mastering core and functional fitness. For example, you are more likely to successfully train for a 10K after you've effectively learned how to engage your core and can physically move throughout your day without pain. Imagine having to go out for a four-mile training run after your back has been mildly aching or having to worry that you may leak urine once you get past mile two. In my experience, focusing on "fitness" becomes a bigger piece of the pie the further you move into motherhood.

I can't tell you how long it will take to reach the top of the CFF pyramid, and as you saw from my back injury story, there's no guarantee you'll stay there. But that's part of the process. You can get to the top, step away, and return to the top stronger. As your motivation, consistency, challenges, stage of motherhood, and exercise program change, so will your place on the pyramid (or the percentages components make up on the pie chart). The flexibility of the CFF framework helps you adjust your priorities and stay consistent, no matter what stage you're in. You'll avoid feelings of failure and frustration, and you won't ever have to start over. If you're like many moms and feel overwhelmed trying to balance fitness with everything else, the CFF approach will simplify things for you. By focusing on what matters most (core, function, or fitness), you can put your energy where it's needed, without feeling pressure to do everything at once. This is how you keep moving forward. (See Appendix B for more details on the CFF framework.)

Take Action

Let's take a moment to reflect on the ten benefits of strength training. Choose one of the following to think about:

1. Which benefits feel most meaningful to you at this stage of motherhood? Let those serve as your personal motivators as you commit to movement.
2. How do these benefits support the kind of lifestyle you want to build, physically, emotionally, or as a role model? Keep that vision in mind as you move forward.

3

Figuring Out What You Need

> *Key Insights from This Chapter*
>
> 1. While global health organizations provide general physical activity guidelines for health, you need to translate those recommendations into an individualized plan.
> 2. Self-assessment is one of the first steps in creating a personalized exercise program, but it's not one-and-done. You should reassess your needs and stage of motherhood change.

Organizations like the American College of Sports Medicine (ACSM), the World Health Organization, and the American Heart Association collaborate with medical, public health, and exercise science experts to develop physical activity guidelines. These guidelines outline the minimum recommended activity levels and types of exercise needed to support overall health and reduce the risk of disease. Guidelines may vary based on population and region. Still, there is a consensus globally that adults aim for at least 150 minutes of moderate-intensity aerobic exercise or 75 minutes of vigorous activity per week, along with muscle-strengthening activities on two or more days. While the core recommendations are fairly consistent worldwide, individual adaptations are encouraged to best suit personal health, fitness levels, and circumstances. In my twenty-plus years of working with individuals, I know that true personalization isn't obvious to most people. Despite exercise recommendations being stated as simply as possible, determining how to accomplish them can be difficult.

One of the most important processes I implemented at the Active Mom Fitness Studio was the first-session Prenatal/Postpartum Screening and Consultation. This session is so powerful that I even created an American Council on Exercise-Approved continuing education course for fitness professionals on it (see Appendix B if you're a fitness professional looking for course information). If you and I were in this session, we'd spend an hour discussing and evaluating your exercise and medical history, pregnancy/delivery experience, and areas of wellness like sleep and nutrition. I'd assess your functional movement quality, determine if you need referrals to a healthcare provider, and together we'd narrow down two areas to prioritize as a starting point. Most moms can't remember the last time they received that much attention and find it extremely valuable! So, your next step in the Active Mom journey is to self-assess. By the end of this chapter, you'll understand what your body needs right now and will have identified factors to consider when creating or selecting an exercise plan. And notice I say "plan." With so many options, it's easy to jump around from class to class or select workouts based on duration or music. Although the variety can be fun, choosing random workouts most likely means you're not progressively challenging yourself, not structuring your recovery so your muscles can get stronger, and not meeting your personal needs.

This assessment won't give you a score or generate a workout, but it should give you a perspective that allows you to move through the rest of this book and the fitness world with a personal lens. Please don't write in your book, as you'll want to use this assessment to reevaluate your needs at different stages of motherhood or as your life changes (see Appendix B for a downloadable version of this assessment).

Assessment One

Choose the answer that sounds like you most. After your response, read the considerations below the question.

1. When it comes to strength training, I am:

A. a novice, a beginner, or have never worked out without following an instructor.

B. experienced and confident in my technique with the majority of exercises.

If you've identified as a novice, then learning the proper form for the major movement patterns is an essential starting point. Keep in mind that if your core is weak or you have mobility limitations, it may be difficult to achieve optimal technique, in which case, core strength and mobility should be your priority. You'll want to pay attention to the pace of your workouts. Initially, you'll want to avoid fast-paced formats so that you can take the time needed to ensure proper technique. If you're not being guided by a personal trainer or group exercise instructor, make sure to check your form in a mirror or record yourself performing movements during home workouts.

If you are experienced and confident in your technique performing squats, lunges, rows, chest press, etc., that doesn't mean there isn't room for improvement. To ensure you're getting the most from your workouts, turn your focus to making sure you're using the right muscles at the right time. For example, are your squats quad-dominant or do you use your glutes too? Do you engage your core before performing a push-up?

2. I'd describe my consistency/frequency of exercise as being closest to:

A. consistent. I've exercised consistently for at least one month, meeting aerobic and resistance training guidelines.

B. inconsistent. I have not been exercising consistently, and I perform fewer than two workouts per week. Additionally, choose this response if you're coming back from a long break or have never really exercised before.

If you've been exercising consistently and are currently meeting physical activity guidelines, ask yourself whether you're content with your current activity level and if the frequency, duration, and type of exercise are aligned with your needs and goals at this stage of motherhood. If you decide to make changes, pay attention to the progressions and regressions mentioned in future chapters.

If you haven't been exercising consistently, let's figure out why. You should first determine what your barriers are and begin to consider realistic ways to overcome them. Before any action can occur, you need to be aware of your obstacles and confident in your solutions. Being new to exercise can feel overwhelming but remember a lifetime of physical activity doesn't happen all at once. It's OK to start small and if you want physical activity to be sustainable, it has to work for you.

3. When I'm going through the day or participating in exercise or physical activity, I:

A. move well, with little to no pain or discomfort.

B. often feel sore, tight, or uncomfortable. I don't move the way I used to.

If you move well, this usually indicates that you don't have any major weaknesses or deficits impacting your movement. Keep in mind that if you move well throughout your day but haven't been exercising, you may experience some soreness and discomfort when beginning an exercise routine until your body adapts.

If you have discomfort throughout the day, it will be important for you to identify the cause. Are muscles too tight? Too weak? Do your posture or daily habits need to improve? You should also note whether you're describing pain or limited by an unaddressed injury or undiagnosed condition. If the discomfort is interfering with your quality of life, you're going to want to start at either the "core" or "function" layer of the pyramid, but I'd also encourage you to see a healthcare provider, so your treatment can align with your exercise program.

4. Thinking about the environment in which I'll exercise, I:

A. have access to a variety of appropriate exercise equipment either at home or at the gym.

B. don't have access to much exercise equipment and don't plan to buy any or go to the gym.

If you have access to equipment, this gives you the benefit of variation in your routine and possibly the ability to increase resistance or level of challenge. However, don't always assume heavier is better, or that changing up your exercises each workout is beneficial. For example, many exercise programs designed to increase strength or definition require you to be consistent in your routine for six to twelve weeks. You'll learn in later chapters that increasing resistance isn't the only way to add challenge to your program, so although more equipment can be beneficial, when and how you choose to take advantage of the variety is important.

If you don't have access to equipment, that doesn't mean your workouts are less effective as long as you manipulate other variables to increase challenge. You'll have to be deliberate in your planning so that you're using recovery time, number of sets/reps, range of motion, and tempo to continue to see results. Don't let a lack of equipment get in the way of home workouts. I've worked with many moms who didn't have a choice but to work out at home, and we manipulated those variables so that they continued to make progress.

5. Life can feel unpredictable, but in general, I:

A. have a fairly flexible daily schedule. Even though my days are full, I can find free time and fill it with exercise if I choose.

B. have a pretty set schedule. I have fixed times that can't be altered and very little wiggle room to spontaneously add events to my day.

If you have a flexible schedule, you may have more opportunities to find time for physical activity and have the benefit of rescheduling a workout if you miss the time you originally planned. However, this can backfire if you make assumptions that you'll be able to fit your workout in at some point, distractions and unexpected occurrences, and sabotage your workout intentions. Consider scheduling your workouts if you're often getting to the end of the day realizing your to-do list was too long and you didn't get a chance to exercise.

If your schedule is pretty fixed, this may seem like a disadvantage, but it can be positive to be forced to set a specific time to exercise. Finding a time block for exercise within your routine and sticking to it will give you the best chance of consistency. You may find it harder to attend group classes at specific times, so consider home options. This also means you must hold yourself accountable because more often than not, if you miss your set time, you won't find another time to make up for it.

6. At this stage of mom life, I'd say I lead a/an:

A. active lifestyle. My social activities often include movement, and on the weekends I'm active with my family. My job keeps me on my feet, and I'm the type of person to take the stairs whenever I get the chance.

B. sedentary lifestyle. On the weekends or most evenings, I catch up on my favorite shows or choose social activities like going out to dinner or coffee dates. Time with my children tends toward sitting to play games, doing puzzles, or building Legos, but it would be rare for me to go on a bike ride with my family. Additionally, choose this option even if you fit a workout in each day but still spend much of the day sitting.

If you have an active lifestyle, this is great news when it comes to health. We know that inactivity has an array of adverse health effects. However, if you lead an active lifestyle, consider whether your exercise routine complements it. If you're on your feet all day at work, then moderate to vigorous workouts at night may feel like a struggle, especially if you're pregnant. If you take long walks every day with your newborn, core training might be the only additional activity that you should aim to accomplish at this stage.

If you have a sedentary lifestyle, before focusing too much on structured workouts, it may be more appropriate to aim to move intermittently throughout the day to break up the sedentary behavior. That's not to say you shouldn't incorporate structured workouts, but if you are concerned about your health, a beneficial goal might be just to reduce the amount of time you're not moving, as there might be an increased risk of disease with increased sitting time.[1] Even a few minutes of stretching between calls can reduce stiffness, and a short walk in the late afternoon might improve your ability to think and boost your energy.

That concludes assessment one. Your answers to these questions should have provided you with insight into how confident you feel in your fitness abilities, what might be holding you back from being consistent, and how your body is responding to movement right now. With this perspective, you can make informed decisions about where to start, what to prioritize, and how to adjust your workouts to fit your life as a mom.

Assessment Two

This next section focuses on factors contributing to your physical and mental wellness. For each area, rate yourself on a scale from 1 to 10, where 10 means, "I'm doing great in this area and couldn't improve much even if I tried," and 1 means, "This is a real challenge for me, and I'm struggling." Remember, these ratings are intentionally subjective and based on how you feel about each area, not on any external standard.

- Nutrition
- Sleep (if you're not getting at least five-hour stretches, your rating should be below 5)
- Water intake
- Stress management

All these factors play a crucial role in your fitness journey. I'd hate to see you invest time and effort into exercise without having the lifestyle habits that truly support your progress. Regardless of your fitness goals, how many weeks pregnant you are, or what stage of postpartum you're in, things like nutrition, sleep, hydration, and stress management directly affect your energy levels, weight management, workout performance, and tissue healing.

Take a moment to identify the two areas you rated the lowest. If either of them scored below a 6, pause and ask yourself if that rating is accurate or if you are being overly critical. If you still feel those areas could hold you back from reaching your fitness goals, spend some time brainstorming realistic ways to make improvements. Small changes can have a big impact, and addressing these areas will help you get the most out of your workouts.

I understand that sleep can be unpredictable, especially during pregnancy with the frequent need to use the bathroom or postpartum while meeting the demands of caring for a newborn. If sleep is one of the two priorities you identified, you may not have a solution to get more hours that are within your control. Still, you can factor this information into the intensity and timing of your workouts, or on some days, whether a nap would do you more good than exercise. I will say that sometimes, as moms, we accept that we won't get enough sleep, so we give up on trying to improve our quality of sleep. Behaviors that are negatively associated with sleep include going to bed hungry or thirsty (I had to keep crackers by my bed while pregnant and breastfeeding to ease middle-of-the-night hunger), not getting exposure to sunlight during the day, using the bed for activities other than sleep and sex, not having enough time to relax before bed, and sleeping on an uncomfortable mattress or pillows.[2] So don't give up on addressing sleep as a barrier until you assess habits that can improve sleep quality.

Assessment Three

This assessment helps you identify common obstacles that can make starting or sticking with an exercise routine challenging. I hope that by recognizing these barriers and acknowledging they're not just excuses, you'll feel empowered to develop strategies to overcome them. As with any other obstacle, finding a way to get around it may take some time. Spend time not just identifying your challenges but also pinpointing specifically how they show up in your life. Remember, the goal is to find solutions, so you need to be as precise as possible.

- **Fear.** This can be fear of miscarriage, fear of harm to the fetus, or fear of doing too much too soon after a C-section. This might include fear of your inability to keep up in a class, fear of reinjury, or fear you'll fail. Select fear as a barrier if it's impacting your ability to start or stay consistent with an exercise program.

- **Society.** This might refer to the people in your life or inner circle or people you follow on social media. Influences like cultural trends or religious beliefs also fall into this category. Are you in a family that says you should "put your feet up" while pregnant? Do you follow influencers who claim to have "bounced back" after having a baby? Does culture or religion influence your attitudes toward exercise? Select society as a barrier if external factors or people influence your fitness decisions.

- **Comfort in your body.** Being comfortable in and with your body is more than what your body looks like. Comfort is attending a fitness class and not feeling like you need to hide in the back. Comfort is the ability to accept that you will gain weight during pregnancy. Think about the level of comfort with your body before motherhood. Have you struggled with body image? What do you think when you see yourself in the mirror every day? Are you a former athlete discouraged by your current lack of athleticism? Select comfort as a challenge if you have or have had recurring negative thoughts about your body.

- **Low energy level.** Most of us can think of plenty of times when we've been able to push past fatigue to meet a work deadline or to cram for an exam in college. After a late night out in your early twenties, getting up for work was somehow manageable. Or maybe you've pushed through a cold that had you run down. Your hormones during pregnancy, the lack of sleep postpartum, and the mental energy of parenting are not that type of tired. It's a type of tiredness that, at times, you can't and shouldn't push through. Does the first trimester have you struggling to keep your eyes open at dinner? Is your child teething and waking you up several times during the night? Are you balancing a promotion and weekends tied up in your kid's activities? Select low energy as a barrier if you're frequently fatigued or in a cycle of low energy that impacts your quality of life and motivation to work out.

- **All-or-none mentality.** For some goals, like reading more books or cleaning out a closet, we tend to accept incremental steps like reading a few pages every night or starting by just choosing clothes to donate. But for whatever reason, when it comes to goals like weight loss or eating healthier, people tend to have the all-or-none mentality. Are you someone who misses a workout and then, in turn, it derails your nutrition? Do you get frustrated with missing a few workouts and then feel like you need an entirely new plan? If life feels too busy, do you tell yourself that you'll get back to the gym when things calm down? If you planned a thirty-minute walk during lunch, but a meeting runs over fifteen minutes, do you forego the remaining fifteen minutes and skip the walk? Select the all-or-none mentality as an obstacle if anything less than perfection hinders building your fitness foundation.

- **Pain.** Whether it be discomfort related to pregnancy or childbirth, years of chronic pain, or an acute injury, pain has physical and emotional repercussions. Do you suffer from frequent pain in your hips, back, or wrists? Have you been Have you struggled to stay consistent with physical therapy and still feel occasional flare-ups or discomfort from your injury?" Did you deal with SI joint pain during pregnancy and now fear aggravating it? Select this barrier if current or past pain interferes with or is triggered by physical activity.

- **Lack of support.** Support can take many forms and impact your activity in various ways. Health education is a form of support that helps us make informed decisions. Childcare is a form of support that allows us time for healthy behaviors. Our friends, family, and partners can inspire and encourage us to be active or make us feel bad about our changing bodies and unmotivated to exercise. Has your healthcare provider encouraged you to exercise? Do you belong to a gym with daycare? Are your friends physically active? Does your family comment on your weight? Does your partner make fitness feel like a luxury? Select this barrier if you feel unsupported, and it creates an environment or mindset that makes it hard to make fitness progress.

- **Modified programming.** Modification is a common word used in exercise, but truthfully, I've never liked it. Most would agree that a modification is an adjustment to the standard version of an exercise, like knee push-ups instead of full push-ups. In a group exercise setting, an instructor might provide an exercise modification to someone if they've been injured or aren't at the necessary fitness level. I don't like that modification implies that one version of an exercise is better than the other, and if you can't do the version given, it is a negative. As you go through this book, I hope that your takeaway is that the best version of the exercise is the one that works for you. So, I wonder, do you have trouble getting on and off the floor, so you skip entire sections of your app workouts? Do you have incontinence and avoid certain exercises in your favorite class? Are you pregnant and going to classes that are not prenatal-friendly? It doesn't feel good to consistently participate in workouts that have to be "modified" for you. Select this as a barrier if your current routine or plan involves exercises you can't do or if you're discouraged in classes because you always need modifications.

Now that you've identified obstacles to your fitness success, it's time to troubleshoot. We can't solve everything in this one chapter, and some challenges will require you to dig deep for a remedy. Some barriers may be outside of your control at this point in life, and you may not have a fix, in which case you'll want to make sure to factor that into your goal setting. I'll give you a few examples of this step and then encourage you to spend some time thinking about this portion of the assessment.

Examples: If fatigue is a barrier, your first step could be identifying the time of day when you have the most energy. If you're suffering from a lack of sleep, scheduling a workout closest to the time you wake can be effective. If you don't feel supported by the people in your life, one strategy could be to find an online community of like-minded individuals. If you've identified being uncomfortable in your body as something that might hinder your efforts, consider self-compassion exercises or gaining confidence by tracking small wins.

That concludes the third assessment. Your answers should have provided insight into which lifestyle factors may support or interfere with your fitness progress. You've identified key areas that could be barriers, but more importantly, you've started thinking about realistic solutions. Whether it's improving sleep quality, managing stress more effectively, or making small nutrition and hydration changes, these adjustments will support your workouts and overall well-being. Now, with a clearer understanding of what's working and what needs attention, you can set realistic and achievable goals.

Assessment Fourth (For Expecting Moms)

This last assessment isn't a true assessment but provides information on pre-activity screening during pregnancy. There are few maternal medical conditions where exercise is cautioned against during pregnancy, which is why I didn't lead with a list of contraindications. For moms with a healthy pregnancy, without complications, the benefits of exercise outweigh the risks, even if you haven't been exercising. The conditions in which exercise is not recommended are not caused by exercise. So, for those reasons, I don't like to cause unnecessary fear. If you're pregnant and have not talked to your obstetrician or doctor about exercise, you can use the Get Active Questionnaire for Pregnancy released by the Canadian Society for Exercise Physiology (CSEP).[3] This self-assessment "is designed to identify the small number of individuals who should seek medical advice as a first step to becoming or continuing to be physically active during the months that they are pregnant, and to help the majority of healthy pregnant individuals overcome any concerns they might have with getting or staying active."

You've made it to the end of the assessments. Keep in mind this isn't a one-time exercise. As you transition through different phases of motherhood and life, return to this chapter and reassess your needs.

To illustrate the value of reassessment, I want to share Sheila's story. Not only is she a great example of why reevaluating is important, but she's also been part of Active Mom Fitness since its inception. I've had the privilege of working with her through two postpartum recoveries, a pregnancy, and, most remarkably, a cancer diagnosis, treatment, and survivorship. At every stage, we discussed how much sleep she's getting, her work schedule, her level of comfort, and other supporting and hindering factors in her wellness journey. We shifted her program when her energy was lower, when she went from studio workouts to virtual sessions at home, and when she went from moving pain free to navigating a body that felt unfamiliar.

Despite all these changes, we always returned to her "why," her reason for showing up, and used exercise as a tool to support her needs at that moment. My role was small; she did the work. And Sheila, if you're reading this, I have never been more inspired by anyone. To this day, she remains committed to physical activity for her health, her wellness, and her family, proving that when you adapt fitness to your needs, you can succeed and continue forward.

Take Action

If you felt rushed or didn't have as much time to reflect as you wanted, consider one of the following next steps:

1. Make it tangible. Go to the appendix and photocopy the assessment, so you can write down your answers and refer back to them as you move through the book.
2. Give it space. Take a day or two to reflect on the challenges or barriers you identified. Then return to your list and begin thinking through possible solutions with a fresh perspective.

Part II

4

Your Core from the Inside Out

Key Insights from This Chapter

1. Your core is more than just your abs. It's a system of muscles working together to provide stability, support posture, and adapt to the physical demands of motherhood.

2. The diaphragm, transverse abdominis, and pelvic floor muscles form the foundation of core strength. When these muscles coordinate effectively, they help prevent issues like back pain and bladder leaks.

The core can be visualized as a 360-degree cylinder between your diaphragm and pelvic floor, supporting your spine and pelvis from all sides. It consists of deep and superficial muscles that stabilize your body and manage physical stress, particularly during pregnancy and postpartum.

Before we get into specific muscles, let me provide you with an overview of the role of your core. The muscles that make up your core are responsible for stability when your arms and legs are moving, breathing, helping your body change position and generate force, managing resistance and loads placed on your body, continence, and postural control. In most cases, no single muscle is solely responsible for any role, meaning your core muscles work together. To optimize your core training, you should ensure that the right muscles activate at the right time. Effective core training programs improve the synergy between core muscles. As I go into more detail about specific muscle groups below, you'll learn how to keep your core strong during pregnancy and why the proper core training progression is so important after having a baby.

Prioritize These Muscles

When I train moms, I prioritize three key muscle groups: the diaphragm, transverse abdominis (shortened to TrA), and pelvic floor muscles (PFM). These muscles are your stabilizers, and they work together to provide essential support for your body. Exercises like crunches help us engage the more superficial core muscles, but for moms, it's important that we don't overlook the deeper core muscles. Training the deeper core muscles is about more than building strength. It also focuses on developing a strong mind-body connection, teaching these muscles to work together, and enabling them to activate automatically to support you in everyday movements. In fact, this type of motor control training shows significant reductions in low back pain and disability compared to other forms of exercise or manual therapy. This emphasizes how essential it is for these deeper muscles to function correctly to manage pain and maintain overall mobility and quality of life.[1]

Transverse Abdominis

Wrapping around your trunk like a corset, the transverse abdominis plays a crucial role in stabilizing your spine and pelvis. Keeping this muscle functional can help reduce your risk of low back pain as your body navigates physical changes. As pregnancy progresses, your growing belly and breasts shift your center of gravity forward, placing greater demands on your body. A well-trained transverse abdominis serves as your first line of defense, automatically activating to support you and preventing other muscles from becoming overloaded as they compensate for changes in posture and weight distribution.

Pelvic Floor Muscles

Unfortunately, most of us don't talk much about pelvic floor muscles until pregnancy or postpartum. Likewise, training them doesn't usually become a priority until they aren't functioning as they should. Like the transverse abdominis, PFM play an essential role in core strength and function through motherhood. Pelvic floor muscles can be visualized as a supportive hammock running from the pubic bone to the tailbone, consisting of three layers that work in coordination with the diaphragm and TrA to optimize core stability. These muscles are responsible for functions such as supporting the bladder, bowel, and reproductive organs, maintaining continence, and even contributing to orgasms. Although they usually activate automatically, learning to engage them voluntarily during increased physical demands can help lower the risk of issues like incontinence or prolapse. Stress, trauma, and hormonal changes from pregnancy and childbirth can cause these muscles to weaken or tighten, making it essential for moms to know how to both contract *and* relax them effectively during exercise and core training.

PELVIC FLOOR MUSCLES

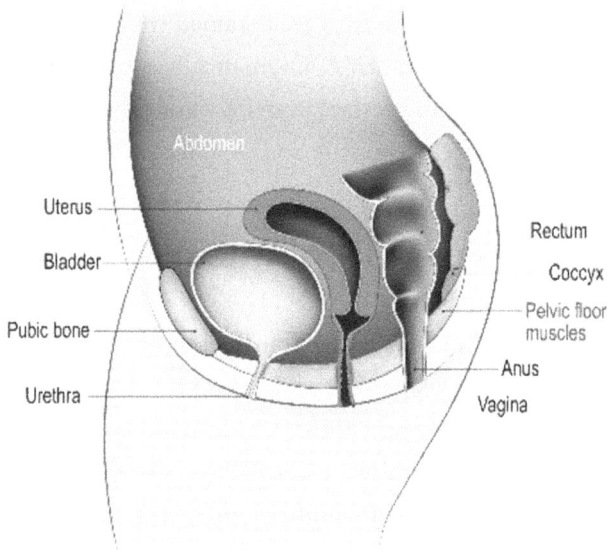

Pelvic floor muscles and abdominal organs. The pelvic floor muscles span from the pubic bone at the front to the tailbone at the back, supporting the abdominal organs and creating the base of the core. © Designua/Adobe Stock. Used under Standard License.

Diaphragm

If you've ever taken a Pilates class, you know that breath is an important part of core training. The diaphragm, a muscle responsible for breathing, also serves as the "ceiling" of the core. When it works in coordination with the TrA and the "basement" of the core, the pelvic floor muscles, it contributes to spinal stability. Yet if the pelvic floor and deep abdominal muscles aren't functioning optimally, or if your baby is taking up more room in the belly, it can alter the way the diaphragm moves, making breathing feel different or more restricted.

How Do These Muscles Coordinate in a Well-Functioning Core?

When you inhale, your diaphragm moves downward, causing the pelvic floor muscles to lengthen downward and the TrA to relax as your belly expands outward. Conversely, as you exhale, the diaphragm lifts, and the pelvic floor muscles and TrA contract, moving upward and inward, respectively. You can imagine the "ceiling" and "basement" muscles moving in harmony with each breath. When this trio of core muscles work together effectively, they increase intra-abdominal pressure (IAP), providing stability for your trunk. Training these muscles can improve automatic co-contraction and function.

A Note on Intra-Abdominal Pressure

Intra-abdominal pressure is the internal pressure within your abdomen and pelvis that helps stabilize your spine.[2] It naturally increases during activities like lifting, coughing, and running to provide support. Think of a plastic water bottle. When the cap is loose, the bottle is soft and easy to squeeze, but when the cap is tightened, the pressure inside makes it more rigid. Your core responds similarly to movement. When your muscles engage properly, IAP increases to help stabilize your body (becoming more rigid).

The intra-abdominal pressure your body generates isn't the same for everyone, even during the same activity. Things like breathing, posture, and core strength all affect how much pressure is created. In fact, some exercises that seem intense may actually put less pressure on your core than everyday movements like lifting a toddler or getting up from a deep couch.[3]

It's not completely clear how higher IAP affects the pelvic floor, but we do know that the amount of pressure, how often it happens, and whether movements are controlled all make a difference. If your pelvic floor is functioning well, exercise can help reinforce its automatic activation. But if there's already some weakness or dysfunction, high-pressure activities might add extra strain and lead to discomfort or symptoms.[4]

During and after pregnancy, your ability to regulate this pressure may change as your core adapts. If you can't manage pressure as effectively, your risk for certain conditions may increase. We'll discuss these in the next chapter.

Bringing It All Together

With an understanding of these three muscle groups and intra-abdominal pressure, you can see how the changes your body goes through during pregnancy and postpartum can affect your core strength, breathing, posture, balance, and even bladder control. Think about how your core engages when you bend down to lift a car seat, push a stroller uphill, or carry your growing baby for extended periods. If your core muscles aren't working efficiently, whether due to changes from pregnancy, a weak core, or a disrupted breathing pattern, you might notice back pain, feel unsteady, or even experience urine or fecal leaks during these routine tasks.

Whether you're new to core training or an experienced exerciser, focusing on deep core strength is essential. Let's start with a simple yet important activity to build that foundation.

Step One—Practice Optimal Breathing (Belly Breathing)

- Set Up: Sit in a chair with your knees bent and feet flat on the floor. Keep your neck and shoulders relaxed.
- Hand Placement: Place one hand on your upper chest and the other on your belly.
- Inhale: Breathe in slowly and deeply through your nose, directing the air toward your belly. The hand on your abdomen should move away from your spine, while the hand on your chest stays relatively still.
- Exhale: Exhale through your mouth, allowing the hand on your belly to move inward toward your spine as you release the breath.

Step Two—Activate the Transverse Abdominis

- Set Up: Stand with your ribcage centered over your hips, neck, and shoulders relaxed.
- Hand Placement: Place your thumbs on your hip bones with your fingers resting below. Slide your thumbs and pointer fingers toward each other until they touch, forming a triangle over your lower abdomen.
- Inhale: Take a slow, deep breath through your nose, directing the air toward your belly. Your thumbs and fingers should separate from each other as you breathe in.
- Exhale and Engage: Exhale through your mouth, drawing your deep abdominal muscles inward toward your spine. Your thumbs and fingers should move back together or overlap slightly if you're achieving a deep contraction. This is where

you should feel your TrA activating. If you're not sure if you're feeling your TrA, place your hands on your lower abdomen and cough forcefully. You'll feel these muscles engage and contract. That is your TrA.

Step Three—Visualize and Engage Your Pelvic Floor Muscles

- Set Up: Stand with feet wider than hip distance apart, hands resting on your hips.
- Inhale and Visualize: Take a deep breath in through your nose. As you inhale, lower into a squat position while imagining the pelvic floor muscles gently expanding and lengthening downward, like a hammock relaxing toward the floor.
- Exhale and Lift: As you exhale through your mouth, rise back up from the squat and visualize lifting the pelvic floor muscles as though drawing them gently upward toward your belly button.

If you're having trouble connecting with your PFM, here are some creative cues that I've heard over the years:

- Imagine you're holding in gas, closing your anus.
- When low in the squat, picture picking up a blueberry off the ground and lifting it upward without squishing it as you come back to standing (gently place it back on the ground when you descend into the squat again).
- Visualize gently sucking a spaghetti noodle up through your vagina.

Now that you understand how to activate and coordinate your transverse abdominis and pelvic floor muscles with your breathing,

I hope you're motivated to incorporate this approach into your core training. Maintaining core function during pregnancy and rebuilding strength postpartum are absolutely possible! I've had clients who were complimented by nurses during delivery for their core strength and ability to change positions with ease. I've also worked with moms who expected to struggle with movement as their pregnancies progressed, yet they remained agile and comfortable all the way to their due dates.

While the core consists of many muscles, some experts count as many as twenty-nine, the coordination of these three (the diaphragm, TrA, and PFM) is especially important for moms. Once you feel confident in your breathwork and coactivation, you can begin incorporating other core muscles, like the obliques, rectus abdominis, multifidus, and erector spinae. Let's take a brief look at the function of these additional muscles.

Multifidus

This back muscle runs along your spine and is another stabilizing muscle that could easily be grouped with the trio we've already prioritized. However, it can be challenging to intentionally engage and feel the multifidus activating without touching it. That is why I didn't incorporate it into our practice activity, but it is essential to strengthen the multifidus for core stability.

Erector Spinae

These back muscles run vertically along each side of your spine as well. They're responsible for trunk extension. For example, when you bend over to tie your shoe, the erector spinae help you stand upright again. If you're familiar with yoga, these muscles also assist in extending backward in poses like cobra.

Obliques

You have both internal and external obliques, with the internal obliques sitting beneath the external obliques. For this book, all you need to remember is that these muscles help your trunk rotate right and left. These are your twisting muscles.

Rectus Abdominis

Most of us can visualize these muscles, as they are the "six-pack" muscles of the abs. They are separated down the midline by a collagen tissue called the linea alba. The main function of your rectus abdominis is spinal flexion. Using the shoe example again, they're the muscles that help you bend forward from a standing position. They're also engaged in movements like crunches and sit-ups, which flex the spine forward.

I hope your takeaway from this chapter is recognizing that core training isn't just about isolated muscles; it's the foundation for movement, strength, and function in motherhood. Whether you're navigating pregnancy, rebuilding postpartum, or years into mom life, prioritizing these deep core muscles will improve how you move, feel, and perform daily tasks (see Appendix B for resources on training the essential core muscles).

Take Action

Choose one of the following to try as you begin building core awareness:

1. Start with the breathing activity introduced in this chapter. Focus on feeling your hands move in the right direction with each breath. Once that feels natural, add pelvic floor engagement. Remember, breathing alone can take time to master, and that's perfectly okay.
2. Review the pelvic floor cues from this chapter and see if you can improve your sense of engagement.

5

It's Not Just You and You Don't Have to Live with It

> *Key Insights from This Chapter*
> 1. Progressing core exercises gradually, based on how your body responds, not how fast you want results, builds strength without overstressing healing tissues.
> 2. Everyday movements like lifting, rolling, and getting out of bed are opportunities to practice breath and core support.

For too long, the changes to a mom's body and the sometimes accompanying conditions have not been widely and transparently discussed. The lack of awareness and conversation has left many moms assuming that pain or incontinence is simply "part of the deal." Often moms are even met with dismissive attitudes like, "Well, you had a baby, so." At the same time, it's understandable why sharing information about symptoms isn't as transparent as maybe it should be because hyperfocusing on possible physical challenges could cause some moms unnecessary worry and stress. As a result, issues like leaking urine when you sneeze or painful sex have become normalized, and many moms have accepted them as an unavoidable and untreatable part of motherhood. This chapter aims to empower you with knowledge and convey that while pregnancy and postpartum conditions are common, more common than many realize, they don't have to be something you just live with. There are resources and strategies to help moms thrive, and this chapter will outline the basics for you.

If You're Experiencing Symptoms

If you're already experiencing the symptoms this chapter describes, it's natural for you to search online for information and reassurance. While it can be comforting to know you're not alone and that solutions exist, diving too deep into blogs and articles can quickly become overwhelming. Instead of hours of research, focus on simplifying your approach in identifying support and solutions. When you're ready to learn more, prioritize resources from qualified physical therapists or research-based studies. Avoid content that uses fear tactics or rigid "do and don't" lists. If you're looking for emotional support, it's OK to talk to a trusted mom friend about her experience, keeping in mind that her body is not your body. However, for true healing and a treatment plan, seek out a professional who specializes in helping moms like you. Your first step should always be getting a referral to a pelvic health or pelvic floor physical therapist from your doctor. If pelvic health physical therapists aren't available in your area, consider virtual programs designed by qualified professionals for your condition. Be sure to ask whether the pelvic floor therapists specialize in pregnancy and postpartum specifically, as not all of them do.

If You Aren't Experiencing Symptoms

Even if you haven't experienced the conditions we'll review, I encourage you to read on so that if they do occur, you won't feel surprised, scared, or ashamed. If you're not dealing with these challenges, please keep your awareness broad and don't go down the rabbit hole of researching worst-case scenarios. Think of it like this: A professional soccer player knows ACL injuries are a risk in her sport. She trains to strengthen key muscles, practices proper movement mechanics, and makes smart choices on the field to lower that risk, but she doesn't avoid playing out of fear or spend hours researching surgeries for an injury she may never get. Instead, she stays informed, takes preventive steps, and trusts that if an issue arises, she'll have the right support and resources to handle it.

Before we dive into the content, I'd like to remind you that my responsibility as an Exercise Physiologist is to design exercise programs that address your unique needs, including consideration for any health condition you may have. While I focus on how these conditions affect movement and how exercise can be a useful tool, I don't diagnose or provide medical treatment plans. If you're experiencing symptoms, I strongly encourage you to consult a healthcare professional. The best approach to health and wellness combines the right exercise program with proper medical care, giving you the support you deserve. With that said, to ensure that this chapter was accurate and up to date, I consulted Dr. Samantha Fazio, a pelvic health physical therapist and owner of Pelvio Physical Therapy, to review the information and provide additional insight based on her years working with the pregnant and postpartum populations.

What Is Diastasis Recti?

Diastasis rectus abdominis (DRA), commonly called abdominal separation, happens when the connective tissue running down the center of your abdomen stretches and weakens. During pregnancy, this tissue called the linea alba stretches due to hormones and your growing baby, so your rectus abdominis muscles (the superficial "six-pack" abs) shift further apart. There is also evidence that obesity, smoking, multiple pregnancies, and diabetes can contribute to abdominal separation in moms.[1]

Diastasis recti can appear anywhere from just below your rib cage to beneath your belly button. It's important to know that your rectus abdominis muscles were never fused, so there's always a small, natural gap between them. Ideally, the stretched tissue returns close to its baseline after you give birth, but for some moms, the separation lingers postpartum, leading to a diagnosis of DRA.

Is DRA Inevitable?

Research consensus on the exact prevalence of diastasis recti doesn't exist due to differences in measurement methods and criteria in diagnosis and evaluation. However, experts agree that nearly all moms experience some degree of abdominal separation by the end of the third trimester. While this percentage decreases over time, studies indicate that 39–45 percent of moms still have DRA at six months postpartum, and up to 33 percent may still experience it at one year postpartum.[2] As you can see, this condition is common from pregnancy through postpartum.

How Does DRA Impact Core Strength and Function?

As you've learned in previous chapters, core function depends on the synergy between core muscles. When abdominal separation occurs, it can disrupt this coordination, making it harder to perform core exercises with the strength and stability you need. While preventing DRA during pregnancy may not be entirely possible, I believe you can choose exercises that help you maintain core control and minimize unnecessary strain on your stretching abdominal wall. Similarly, you're starting with a weaker core postpartum, so focusing on movements that gradually rebuild strength can prevent overloading healing tissues.

Think of the stretched tissue in DRA like you would the stretched ligament in an ankle sprain. In healing from an ankle sprain, you probably understand that you can't completely control your recovery timeline, but you're going to ensure that you don't perform movements that could slow recovery or worsen the injury. You understand that with an ankle sprain, your joint isn't as stable as it should be, and your primary focus is going to be to regain function first in daily life and then in physical activity or exercise. The same principle applies to DRA, the goal is to gradually strengthen the linea alba and abdominal muscles to support overall core function and daily movement.

Exercise Strategies for Diastasis Recti

If you're dealing with DRA after childbirth, targeted core exercises that engage the transverse abdominis and rectus abdominis can help.

While there's no single "gold-standard" approach, many effective programs emphasize pelvic floor activation, proper breathing, and posture work to restore function gradually.[3] Rather than focusing solely on closing the gap, the goal of exercise is to rebuild strength and improve how the abdominal muscles and connective tissue function together. There is no universal approach to DRA exercises, but when I work with moms with DRA, we follow the CFF core training progression, which you'll learn more about in the next chapter. If you have DRA, a key starting point in the core progression is to figure out which positions and movements create the strongest core activation without breath-holding, bearing down, or "sucking in." Here are a few more strategies if you're exercising with DRA or hope to do what's in your control to prevent it:

- **Manage IAP with breath:** Intra-abdominal pressure is not inherently a bad thing. This pressure is necessary to stabilize your body during movements and is created during everyday actions like sneezing, coughing, lifting, and bending. As you've already learned, breathing helps you manage IAP. With DRA, if you exhale on exertion rather than holding your breath, you'll manage the pressure to protect the linea alba. Breathing correctly also activates your deeper abdominal muscles, which aids in stability as you regain function.

- **Select the right exercises:** Building on the concept of IAP, it's helpful to understand that when more stability is needed, more IAP is produced. For example, bench pressing heavier dumbbells requires more pressure than lifting lighter ones, and double-leg lifts often create more pressure than single-leg lifts. Similarly, high-impact exercises may generate more IAP than low-impact ones, and full range-of-motion movements typically need more IAP than shortened ranges of motion.

If you're concerned about DRA, pay attention to which exercises feel most demanding when it comes to stability and core engagement. This awareness can help guide your exercise choices during pregnancy and inform a safe, effective progression postpartum. Ask yourself: Can you breathe through the movement, or do you catch yourself holding your breath? Is it an activity you're familiar with and comes naturally, or is it a new challenge? For instance, if you've been a lifelong runner, a light jog might feel easier to manage than a brisk walk on an incline. Self-assessment and selecting exercises appropriate for you rather than following a dos and don'ts list is key.

- **Progression:** When it comes to rebuilding core strength and function, a progressive approach ensures that exercises are appropriately challenging without overstressing tissues. A gradual progression in exercise allows you to build a solid foundation before moving on to more advanced exercises, ensuring your body can handle each new challenge effectively. An example of this might be you starting to train your core with heel slides, moving on to heel drops, and eventually working your way up to the more challenging dead bug. Signs like bulging, doming, sinking at the midline, or excessive back arching indicate that an exercise may be too challenging for you at this moment.

Daily Life Strategies

Now that you have a basic understanding of diastasis recti and exercise, let's talk about other factors that may play a role in preventing or recovering from abdominal separation. Many of these are theories, with more research hopefully on the horizon.

- **Address Constipation:** Exercise isn't the only thing that increases IAP. Straining during a bowel movement can also increase intra-abdominal pressure. Constipation and straining are quite common during and after pregnancy. If you're pushing and straining during bowel movements, talk to your healthcare provider for support.

- **Focus on Posture:** Pregnancy and postpartum anatomical changes can increase the likelihood of your pelvis tilting or your ribs flaring. Since your abdominal muscles are attached to your ribs, this flaring can keep the abdomen in a stretched position. Aim to keep your ribs stacked over your hips when standing to maintain a more neutral alignment and reduce the lengthening of your abdominal tissues.

- **Exhale When Lifting:** Exhaling during effort or exertion translates outside of the gym as well. Everyday movements, like picking up your child, standing from the couch, rolling over in bed, or getting out of the car, require core stability and increase IAP. To manage this pressure and protect your core, exhale as you lift, rise, or roll like you would if lifting weights.

- **Nourish Your Body:** Adequate intake of nutrients such as protein, vitamin C, and collagen can facilitate tissue recovery. Staying hydrated and eating nutrient-dense foods can support repair, function, and overall recovery.[4]

- **Protect Your Core When Sneezing or Coughing:** Sudden forceful movements like sneezing or coughing create a significant increase in IAP and stress on your core. After a C-section, moms are often given a bolster (or pillow) to press against their abdomen for support when coughing, but this principle applies to all moms. To reduce strain, gently engage your deep core muscles, including your pelvic floor, by drawing and lifting them in before a sneeze or cough, helping to protect your healing abdominal tissues. This is a skill that requires not only strength but also timing and coordination. A pelvic floor physical therapist can help you address any reasons why this might be difficult for you.

What Is Pelvic Floor Muscle Dysfunction?

PFD, pelvic floor dysfunction is a broad term that describes various issues that arise when the muscles of the pelvic floor aren't functioning properly. Pelvic floor dysfunction can cause a range of issues due to weak, tight, or poorly coordinated pelvic muscles. Some common symptoms of pelvic floor dysfunction include the feeling of heaviness in or something protruding from the vagina, difficulty fully emptying the bladder, leaking urine when coughing, laughing, or exercising, frequent or urgent need to urinate, constipation, and pain during sex.[5]

Is PFD Inevitable?

Like many women's health issues, the exact causes of PFD are not fully understood, but factors like pregnancy, childbirth (both vaginal and C-section), menopause, and obesity can weaken or stretch the pelvic muscles. Like DRA, there isn't a consensus on prevalence, which is due to information collection methods and evaluation at various periods of a woman's life, including many studies being done on older women or women who have not had children. I think it's safe to say that PFD is common but not inevitable. A questionnaire was given to 2,000 pregnant and postpartum women, and nearly half of them reported at least one symptom of bladder, bowel, or sexual dysfunction during pregnancy and postpartum through a validated questionnaire. Certain factors, like difficulty contracting the pelvic floor, smoking, high BMI, and being over thirty-five, were associated with a higher likelihood of experiencing symptoms. However, in another study of about 200 women, over 90 percent experienced at least one symptom by late pregnancy, with the most common being constipation.[6] With the subjective nature of symptom reporting and various factors contributing to PFD, whether you will experience symptoms is difficult to predict. However, if we return to our soccer player analogy, we can imagine that the longer she plays soccer, and the less time she spends strength training, the higher the likelihood that an injury or symptoms will occur.

Hypertonic versus Hypotonic Pelvic Floor Muscles

During and after pregnancy, the pelvic floor can either become too loose (hypotonic) or too tight (hypertonic), both of which can contribute to dysfunction. A hypotonic pelvic floor means the muscles are underactive, making it difficult for them to provide adequate support for the bladder and pelvic organs. This can result in leakage during activities that put pressure on the abdomen. On the other hand, a hypertonic pelvic floor occurs when the muscles remain overactive or too tight and struggle to relax fully. This excessive tension can contribute to symptoms like discomfort during intercourse, constipation, or difficulty emptying the bladder. Since these require different treatment strategies, being accurately diagnosed is essential. Some people benefit from pelvic floor strengthening exercises, while others may need to focus on relaxation techniques first. A pelvic floor physical therapist can help assess your muscle function and guide you in choosing the most effective strategies.

What Is Incontinence?

Incontinence is a condition where a person loses control over their bladder or bowel functions. This means they may involuntarily leak urine or stool. Urinary incontinence is one of the most common symptoms of pelvic floor muscle dysfunction.[7] This can show up as stress incontinence, causing urine leakage during activities like coughing, sneezing, or jumping. It can also appear as urge incontinence, causing a sudden, intense need to urinate that may make it difficult to reach the bathroom in time.

What Is Pelvic Organ Prolapse (POP)?

Pelvic organ prolapse (POP) occurs when the pelvic floor muscles or connective tissues supporting the pelvic organs become too weak or stretched, causing the organ to shift from its normal position. This can involve the bladder, uterus, rectum, or top of the vagina descending downward into or even protruding through the vaginal opening. It's important to note that if you see or feel a pelvic organ prolapse, you are not necessarily seeing or feeling the organ itself. The organ will descend into the front or back wall of the vaginal canal. The front or back vaginal wall will then collapse toward the vaginal opening and this is what you will see or feel with a prolapse.

Dr. Samantha uses this analogy to explain prolapse to her patients: Your pelvis and pelvic organs are like a boat sitting at a dock. The dock is your bony pelvic ring, the boat is your bladder/uterus/rectum, the ropes holding the boat to the dock are your fascia and ligaments, and the water is your pelvic floor muscles. If the water goes down or doesn't provide adequate buoyancy, the boat will sink down and there will be greater pull and tension on the ropes. This is how pelvic floor strengthening can help reduce the strain on the ligaments, provide lift support to the organ, reduce symptoms of a prolapse, and reduce pelvic or low back pain. If the water level is perfect, but the ropes are too slack or torn, the boat will not remain in position. This is analogous to how your ligaments and fascia change after vaginal childbirth. No matter how strong your pelvic floor is, sometimes the ligaments can no longer hold the organs in position. This is where you may be recommended to try a pessary (a pelvic organ support tool much like inserting a tampon or NuvaRing) or, ultimately, a surgical repair if the prolapse is severe. A pelvic floor physical therapist can help assess what the issue is (i.e., the ropes or the water) and recommend a course of action that is right for you.

A large study surveying nearly 4,000 women found that those who lifted heavier weights (over 50 kilograms) were actually less likely to report prolapse symptoms than those who lifted lighter weights ($\leq$15 kilograms) or didn't lift at all. In fact, women in the lighter lifting category were twice as likely to experience symptoms of vaginal bulging.[8] Other factors, such as age, history of vaginal births, constipation, or a family history of prolapse, were also linked to a higher likelihood of symptoms. During vaginal birth, your ligaments and fascia have to stretch to allow for the baby to be born. In the immediate postpartum period, your organs will be slightly descended. A true pelvic organ prolapse will be diagnosed either by your medical provider or your pelvic floor physical therapist once enough healing time has occurred. If you receive this diagnosis, there are plenty of ways to manage symptoms and prevent them from getting worse. Surgical repair is not always necessary.

Exercise Tips for Pelvic Floor Health

With proper technique, breathing strategies, and progressive training, moms and moms-to-be can safely engage in strength training. A well-designed program that improves pelvic floor coordination and enhances overall core strength may protect you from PFD. Whether your goal is to strengthen weak muscles or relax tight ones, these tips will help you navigate your fitness routine safely and effectively while supporting your pelvic floor.

- **Focus on Strength and Relaxation:** Healthy pelvic floor muscles should be able to contract and relax. If your pelvic floor is tight, avoid exercises that encourage clenching or holding tension until you can properly relax and contract through the full range of motion. I often see moms do this during glute exercises when the glutes aren't activating properly or during core movements that require more strength than the abs can provide. For weak PFM, isolated strengthening exercises like Kegels can help, though it is important to understand how to do a Kegel properly. A Kegel is the contraction and relaxation of the pelvic floor muscles, much like doing a bicep curl. You need to squeeze and lift all three of your holes (urethra, vagina, and anus) and then completely relax the muscles all the way down and open. While Kegels are great for isolated pelvic floor control and strengthening, it's just as important to build strength through total body dynamic exercises that improve function in everyday activities.

- **Exhale during Exertion:** This isn't the first time, and won't be the last time, I encourage you to learn how to breathe during exertion. Breathing may seem automatic, but how you breathe during exercise makes a difference in your pelvic health. As you know, when you lift, push, or strain, your IAP naturally increases. If you hold your breath or inhale during these moments, the IAP increases further and puts undue stress downward on your PFM, increasing the risk for potential dysfunction.[9] Instead, exhale during the effort portion of the movement or in cases of prolapse, even right before the movement. Whether lifting a toddler, squatting, or pushing a stroller uphill, exhaling will help release and reduce the IAP increases and help engage your pelvic floor and deep core muscles at the right time, ultimately stabilizing your pelvis, spine, and trunk.

- **Incorporate PFM Activation into Strength Workouts:** Unless advised by a physical therapist, you don't need to carve out extra time for isolated pelvic floor exercises. I teach moms how to incorporate pelvic floor muscle training into their existing strength workouts. Movements like squats, lunges, and deadlifts naturally engage these muscles, making them a great way to build strength. To maximize activation, exhale and engage your pelvic floor (Kegel) at the hardest part of the movement (such as standing from a squat) and relax as you return to the starting position. Since positions that challenge gravity tend to elicit a stronger pelvic floor response, exercises that involve standing, bracing, or core stabilization can further enhance both strength and function. By applying these techniques, you can strengthen your pelvic floor without adding extra exercises to your routine. If you have a hypertonic pelvic floor, focus on relaxing the pelvic floor muscles between reps or incorporating relaxation poses into your cooldown. Belly breathing is a great way to help your pelvic floor muscles relax.

- **Prioritize Recovery:** After a long day on your feet, it can be helpful to allow your pelvic floor muscles to recover, as they can fatigue just like any other muscle group. Incorporating relaxation techniques into your evening routine can help release tension. While specific studies linking these exact practices to pelvic floor recovery are limited, outcomes that exist are promising. It can be inferred that the general principle of muscle recovery through relaxation and gentle stretching can apply to PFM health as well.

- **Be Cautious with High-Impact Exercises:** High-impact exercises like running and jumping put extra stress on your pelvic floor. For moms with a well-functioning pelvic floor (the muscles act like a trampoline, reflexively contracting before moments of increased pressure to support your organs), physical activity likely has a positive training effect and will continue to promote unconscious pelvic floor muscle co-contraction. However, some moms can lose some of that automatic PFM response during childbirth and don't feel connected to their core muscles after having a baby. If you have pelvic floor dysfunction, high-impact exercise may lead to increased strain or worsening symptoms because your PFM aren't lifting reflexively before impact to support the organs.[10] If that sounds like you, prioritizing strength and control until your body begins responding reflexively to high impact again is essential.

Daily Life Considerations and Strategies for Pelvic Floor Health

Your daily habits and behaviors play a significant role in supporting your pelvic floor health. By being aware of how your everyday activities affect your pelvic floor, you can make small adjustments that support long-term strength and function. Here are some key considerations and strategies to keep in mind as you go about your day.

- **Prevent Constipation:** Chronic constipation or straining with bowel movements can injure the pelvic floor, increasing the risk of dysfunction. To support bowel health, ensure you consume at least 25–30 grams of fiber,[11] stay hydrated, and establish regular bathroom habits. If constipation persists, seek guidance from a healthcare provider to prevent unnecessary pressure on pelvic structures.[12]

- **Manage Weight:** Whether due to weight gain during or after pregnancy or daily activities like wearing your baby, added weight can put extra stress on your pelvic floor. If you have PFD, be aware of the weight you're lifting and how often you're carrying your baby. Although I love the idea of the community and convenience in Mommy and Me exercise classes, if your pelvic floor is weak, I advise against exercising with the additional weight of holding your baby. This applies to babywearing on walks as well. Consider using a stroller instead until you rebuild strength.

- **Improve Mental Health:** Recent research highlights a strong link between pelvic floor disorders and mental health, particularly anxiety and depression. Women with urinary incontinence, pelvic organ prolapse, and fecal incontinence experience significantly higher rates of anxiety and depression than the general population. While the exact relationship isn't fully understood, the emotional toll of pelvic floor dysfunction may contribute to mental health challenges.[13] In the other direction, high stress and anxiety may contribute to or cause pelvic floor dysfunction. Much like the jaw, we tend to clench our pelvic floor muscles when stressed, anxious, or nervous. Chronic clenching or overactivation can lead to hypertonic pelvic floor dysfunction. This underscores the importance of prioritizing stress management in your daily life. By incorporating deep breathing, mindfulness, and restorative movements, you can help calm your nervous system and promote pelvic floor relaxation. If stress or anxiety is a major factor, seeking support through therapy may be beneficial.

- **Track Hormonal Influence.** Hormonal fluctuations can impact symptoms of incontinence, pain, and heaviness, especially during the early menstrual phase. These shifts may affect neuromuscular control and tissue elasticity, leading to increased discomfort and functional changes in the pelvic structures.[14] I've worked with many moms who experienced cyclical prolapse sensations, and we would adjust their exercise program to reduce plyometrics or resistance during that time. Since hormonal fluctuations during the menstrual cycle can worsen pelvic floor symptoms, similar effects may be experienced during various stages of your life as hormones shift. Tracking these patterns can help you better understand your body's responses and make informed modifications to movement, recovery, and self-care.

Understanding Back Pain and Pelvic Girdle Pain

Back pain and pelvic girdle pain (PGP) are common complaints during pregnancy and postpartum, affecting everything from mobility to sleep quality. Back and PGP during pregnancy often result from a combination of physiological, hormonal, and structural changes.

Increased ligament laxity shifts in the body's center of gravity, muscle stretching, and excess weight gain all contribute to added stress on the spine and surrounding muscles. As pregnancy progresses, the growing uterus exerts pressure on nerves and blood vessels, which may also explain why pain tends to worsen in the third trimester. Other factors such as maternal age, previous pregnancies, and preexisting musculoskeletal conditions can also increase the risk.[15]

Pelvic girdle pain is a specific form of pain that affects the joints of the pelvis, including the sacroiliac (SI) joints and the pubic symphysis (front pubic bone). It can cause discomfort in the lower back, hips, groin, or thighs and may be aggravated by movement. Symphysis pubis dysfunction (SPD) is a specific condition that is characterized by excessive movement or instability of the pubic symphysis joint, often causing sharp pain in the front of the pelvis and groin.

Is Pain Inevitable during Pregnancy?

Usually, when working with moms during pregnancy, I would start the session by asking how they felt. I can't tell you the number of times a mom would express that she was feeling good but make the disclaimer that she knows at some point that will change. Many moms anticipate that at some point they will suffer from back pain. While it's true that back pain is common, affecting about 40 percent of expecting moms at some point during pregnancy, it's not inevitable. In fact, most moms I worked with did not experience back pain severe enough to complain, affect daily life, or require exercise modifications.[16] I'd argue that a consistent core and strength training program can lower the likelihood of experiencing back pain. While the research doesn't fully confirm this claim, studies do show that exercise can significantly reduce its severity.[17] However, since many studies do not examine specific core and strength training protocols and research on pregnant people is so limited, I don't think it's accurate to conclude that exercise does not play a preventative role. So, while there are no guarantees, I highly recommend following a strength and core training program to improve your chances of a more comfortable pregnancy.

Pain Postpartum

Back pain and PGP don't always disappear after delivery. Studies show that about one-third of women who had back pain during pregnancy still experience it one year postpartum. The pelvis expands to accommodate birth, but it doesn't automatically "snap back" into place after delivery. Some women experience lingering instability in the sacroiliac joints or pubic symphysis, leading to pain with walking, standing, or uneven weight-bearing.

Pain may also emerge for the first time postpartum, particularly around three to six months after birth. The postpartum period is a perfect storm of muscle weakness, repetitive stress, and increased physical demands. Birth trauma and returning to vigorous physical activity too soon can also play a role in new back and pelvic pain postpartum. Fortunately, there is evidence to show that moms who follow a structured postpartum strength and core training program experience significantly less pain than those who remain inactive.[18]

One of my biggest supporters in writing this book was a client of mine. She came to train with me because she was suffering from back pain. Her son was around two or three, which is an extremely physical time for moms. At this age, your child may still ask to be held or need to be carried up the stairs after falling asleep in the car. You're still lugging strollers and trying to keep your balance centered while getting your arm tugged on because they're trying to escape your grip. I knew with mobility, deep core exercises, and perfecting the deadlift, she could enjoy time with her son without pain. Although it didn't happen overnight, she committed to a progressive exercise program and built her confidence and strength. In fact, I ran into her at the pediatric dentist's office about a year after ending our training sessions together, and she was still exercising and feeling good!

Exercise Tips for Reducing Pain

Physical activity can make a noticeable difference in how your body feels during and after pregnancy . . . and beyond. Staying active appears to minimize some of the biomechanical changes that come with becoming a mother, and exercise can help take pressure off your spine, improve joint stability, and support better posture and alignment. Exercise may also help your body become less sensitive to pain over time. Since back and pelvic pain can impact daily life, mood, and even the ability to work, exercise is an effective way to manage symptoms.[19] Consider these exercise tips and strategies:

- **Form Check:** Exercises like squats, deadlifts, bird dogs, and push-ups all have the potential to cause back pain. These movements require core engagement and if your core muscles aren't working together effectively or aren't strong enough, the spine takes on more of the load than it should. This can lead to excessive arching in the lower back and the risk of injury. To avoid these problems, you can monitor your technique. Observe whether your range of motion (depth) during squats results in needing to overly arch your lower back. When deadlifting, ensure that you're leading the movement by pressing your hips back and hinging from your hips and not your mid-back. Also, ensure that if you're holding a barbell or dumbbells, they almost graze your shins rather than hanging far from your body and pulling on your back. During bodyweight exercises like bird dogs and push-ups, watch to make sure your hips aren't sagging and that your core is stable, preventing an excessive curve in your low back.

- **Focus on Your Deep Core:** As we discussed earlier, the transverse abdominis acts like a corset, stabilizing your spine. Strengthening these deep abdominal muscles creates your own built-in back brace. It's worth noting that combining pelvic floor exercises with deep abdominal muscle exercises is more effective than pelvic floor training done alone. One study showed that after twelve weeks of integrated training, women experienced significant improvements in bladder control, daily function, and emotional well-being. If you're experiencing pain and PFD, a combination training program is your best bet.

- **Find Your Way:** Although certain movements are more likely than others to cause pain for moms with SPD, you shouldn't make assumptions about what you should and shouldn't do. For example, side-lying leg lifts can cause pain for many moms as the leg moves away from the body; however, I worked with a mom who was able to do that movement with no pain just by pointing her toes toward the ground while lifting her leg. I've also seen moms experience increased pain with step-ups, but performing step-downs was not a problem. My point is, don't push through the pain, but do take the time to experiment with variations of exercises, so you can decide what is comfortable for you.

Daily Life Considerations and Strategies

I worked with a mom who suffered from pretty intense pubic symphysis pain after having her daughter. I collaborated with her pelvic floor physical therapist not just in identifying the right strength exercises for her, but we also had to identify daily movements and postures that increased pain. Transparently, this took some time because the increased pain wasn't always in the moment. We'd often have to wait until the end of the day, and if she was in increased pain at night, we'd have to review what she did that day. Although a bit tedious, it was worth it. We learned that sitting in bed working on her laptop was not good for her. Unfortunately, holding her daughter on her lap also increased pain. So, if you're experiencing back or pelvic girdle pain, here are areas of daily life to be mindful of.

- **Posture Awareness:** First, let me remind you that the core is like a cylinder. If you were looking down at someone from the top of their head to the ground, you can visualize the center of the cylinder going through the rib cage and the pelvis. Three common mom postures change the cylinder alignment and possibly lead to increased pain or interfere with your recovery. In the first, you can imagine looking down at a mom and maybe their shoulders are rounded forward, causing their rib cage to round down and possibly their pelvis to be tucked under, giving the flat glute appearance. The other common posture is continuing to hold the increased arch in your low back from pregnancy and sticking your rib cage out. The last usually happens when you are holding a child or a purse or bag on one side. You might find yourself jutting your hip to one side, again disrupting the cylinder.

I'm not saying to strive for a perfect posture or that there even is a perfect posture given everyone's anatomical differences, but you should be mindful of sitting or standing in postures that make it harder for muscles like the glutes or core to activate, postures that impact breathing, or postures that keep tissues and muscles lengthened when they shouldn't be. To start simple, when standing, aim to keep your weight evenly distributed between both of your feet and your rib cage stacked over your hips. When sitting on the couch, avoid always leaning to the same side. When in a chair, aim to keep your knees at hip height and feet flat on the floor. You may also feel more comfortable using a pillow or a rolled towel behind your back when watching TV, working, or riding in a car.

- **Stroller Handling:** People come in all sizes, yet most strollers don't. If you're experiencing pain, especially on days that you take your child for walks, examine how you're handling your stroller. If possible, adjust the handles to a proper height to avoid hunching. Before putting a stroller on your registry, consider choosing one with adjustable handles or going to a store to try it in person. When pushing the stroller on an incline, try lightly engaging your deep abdominal muscles for added stability. Lastly, don't forget to exhale on exertion when lifting your stroller into your car trunk, and bend at your knees when unbuckling your child to get out of the stroller.

- **Lifting Technique:** Most moms have been told to bend at their knees when lifting, and this can be protective when it's feasible. However, in situations where squatting isn't an option, like when you lift your baby from the crib, you should consider the lift more like a deadlift. This means hinging from your hips and using your glutes and hamstrings to support your back. Additionally, pay attention to where the object or your baby is relative to your body before picking them up. For the least amount of stress on your spine or pelvis, ensure your child is close to your body and avoid lifting while twisting by ensuring the object is directly in front of you. If your baby is on the other side of the crib, slide them toward you before lifting them out.

- **Keep Your Legs Closed:** That's right, but it doesn't mean what you think. If you get sharp pains in your pubic bone, you're going to want to slow down some of your movements and avoid separating your legs. In daily life, this might look like sliding both legs together before sitting up and getting out of bed or sitting down to put on your pants or socks. When going on walks, you might find it more comfortable to shorten your steps, and some moms place a garbage bag on their car seat to make it easier to slide both legs out of the door at the same time.

How Much to Share with Your Personal Trainer

I recognize that not all of you will feel confident following an app or designing your exercise program if you're experiencing these common conditions. You may elect to work with a personal trainer or fitness professional as you move from physical therapy back into traditional exercise. I'm not going to tell you that having a conversation about your symptoms is always going to be comfortable or easy, but I am going to encourage you to do it anyway. One of the benefits of working with an exercise professional is that they should be able to customize a program that meets your needs and goals and takes into account any physical limitations or barriers. It's unfair to them if you don't give them the chance to do this for you, but more importantly, it's unfair to you, as you are investing time and money in this person expecting results. As I've already mentioned, the fitness industry still has some work to do when it comes to maternal exercise, so in this next section, I want to give you some guidance to help you identify the right person to work with you and help you manage your pregnancy- or postpartum-related condition. Much of this advice can also apply when choosing an app to follow because no matter where the support comes from, the person providing it or designing it should have the experience and credentials to work with moms like you. Or be willing to have a conversation with you so that you can share what you've learned in this book and work together to come up with the best program possible.

Mary

Before we get to the guidance, let me tell you about Mary. I loved my first job out of college. I was a Fitness Specialist at a corporate fitness center. As part of my role, I taught a boot camp class at lunch. As most boot camps were at the time, this class was high intensity and included high-impact exercises. As a group of regulars formed, I got to know a bit about each participant personally and, of course, became skilled at making recommendations in class based on their fitness levels. A woman named Mary was a part of this group, and I noticed that every time we would do jumping exercises, Mary would opt for a low-impact version like step-outs instead. She eventually shared with me that she was a mom of three and peed every time she jumped. She was completely content performing modifications, and I didn't object. To keep things interesting, I'd get creative and come prepared with new exercises that Mary could do comfortably. However, looking back, I could have done more. I didn't do anything wrong, as pelvic floor

PT was not as widely available or comprehensive as it is today, and none of my gold-standard certifications prepped me to address core conditions like incontinence. But, today, because fitness professionals have more access to research, specialized training, and more referral sources, if your trainer simply modifies for incontinence like I did for Mary, they might not be the best person for you. As an Exercise Physiologist, it isn't within my scope to treat or diagnose incontinence, but I should be capable of prescribing exercises that align with treatment and promote improvement. If Mary were in my class today, I'd refer her to my network of pelvic floor physical therapists, and rather than suggesting low-impact modifications while others were jumping, I might teach her how to engage her pelvic floor right before landing or provide her with a deep core exercise to do.

I shared that story to illustrate that even a highly qualified exercise professional may not be qualified to work with you during your phase of motherhood. Specializing in mom fitness is more than just modifications. You want to work with someone who understands the changes your body goes through and feels confident in choosing exercises that challenge you and support your needs. In addition to science, which involves anatomy, physiology, and the principles of effective and safe exercise programming, you also want a personal trainer who has mastered the art of coaching moms. What I mean by this is the ability to validate your concerns, address your barriers, and motivate you. So, whether evaluating an instructor on an app or a personal trainer at your gym, please take the time to consider the following.

Is There a Way to Be Assessed?

Question to Ask: "How Do You Assess My Current Fitness Level and Adapt My Program as My Needs Change?"

Your trainer should establish a baseline in strength, aerobic capacity, and mobility, while also gathering information about your exercise history, pregnancy/postpartum history, preferences, needs, and any injuries. Your trainer should personalize your program based on this discussion and evaluation and be willing to adapt as your needs change through motherhood or as your fitness priorities evolve. If you're following a program and can't speak to the instructor directly, there should be clear instructions on how to self-assess to determine if the workout intensity or style works for you. You should have information on whether you'll be able to follow the entirety of the program despite having a knee injury, for example, or know whether the format is progressive, so you can gradually return to aerobic activity.

Stage of Motherhood

Question to Ask: "How Do You Adapt My Workouts Throughout Each Trimester?" or "I'm 12 Weeks Postpartum, What Type of Workouts Will We Be Doing?"

Your trainer should not generalize exercises based solely on your stage of motherhood. Instead, they should consider ability and individual factors like energy, discomfort, and sleep. Be wary of instructors who claim they can "fix" or "repair." Unless your trainer is also a medical professional, treating your condition is outside of their scope of practice. Additionally, watch out for overuse of modifications. If you're attending a class and the instructor is constantly providing you with modifications to what the rest of the class is doing rather than having planned exercises specifically appropriate for you, it's probably not the class for you. If you're following an online program and not able to interact with the instructor, the program should include sufficient instructions and cues, along with diverse options to meet your needs. For example, if the exercise being taught is lunges and lunging causes you pain, there should be another option that works the same muscle groups so that you're able to get the same benefit as everyone else using the program (unless of course, you learn so much from this book that you're able to select and substitute your own exercises!).

Credentials

Question to Ask: "What Specific Education or Training Have You Have in Maternal Exercise?"

Ideally, your trainer will have a general certification from reputable organizations like NSCA, ACSM, ACE, or NASM. Additionally, your trainer should have completed courses on prenatal or postpartum fitness and have practical experience working with moms. They should be aware of common symptoms and experiences, like pelvic floor issues and back pain, and understand the impact of symptoms on their exercise routine. The same criteria can be applied to online programs. You should investigate the program's instructors rather than assuming, because the brand is well known, that the instructors are qualified to work with you.

Providing Referrals

Question to Ask: "Have You Worked with Anyone with Diastasis Recti? Are you Comfortable Developing Exercise Programs for Someone with Prolapse?"

A skilled trainer is knowledgeable about core and pelvic floor muscles and can individualize exercise routines with these conditions in mind. Not only should they have basic knowledge, but they should initiate the conversation with you so that they have all the information they need to create a program suitable for you. They should also offer to refer you to a healthcare professional if you indicate any pain or dysfunction or if you're symptomatic and haven't been diagnosed. If possible, find an exercise professional who collaborates with physical therapists or other health professionals to ensure you receive comprehensive care. In an app or online setting, again be wary of fitness programs that claim to treat or fix as a marketing ploy and look for ones that include a progressive approach to core training and encourage you to be under the care of a medical professional.

Avoiding Unrealistic Promises

Question to Ask: "How Long Will It Take for Me to See Results? What Results Can I Expect?"

Your needs and goals should always be heard, but it is the trainer's job to help you assess those goals and provide clear and honest expectations on what it takes to achieve them. A qualified professional will consider all your needs and design a well-rounded program specific to your goals. If your trainer emphasizes aesthetics or postpartum weight loss, or isn't transparent about timelines, then you may want to continue to search for someone with a more holistic approach. The same goes for online programs or AI-generated workouts. Stay away from programs that reinforce the "bounce-back culture," as that is not the reality for most moms.

To wrap up this section, a few other considerations include:

- Convenience: Will you have more success with an at-home virtual program or the gym close to your job?

- Relatability: Do you enjoy spending time with this person, or are you excited to log in?
- Trust: Does this person or program help ease your fears and make you feel confident?

Lastly, remember that a trainer whom you worked with before motherhood may not be the most qualified person to guide you through this new chapter. Prioritize someone who has the expertise you need now.

Take Action

If you're not sure where to start or how to apply what you've learned, consider one of the following next steps:

1. Choose one daily task, like lifting your child, getting off the couch, or climbing stairs, and practice exhaling during the hardest part (exertion). Notice how your core and pelvic floor respond when you do.

2. Spend one day paying attention to how you move. Do you hold your breath when you lift, strain during a bowel movement, or always lean to one side when sitting? Jot down one habit you'd like to adjust and choose a small way to start.

6

Core Training for Moms

Key Insights from This Chapter

1. Progress isn't always linear; knowing when to pause, skip, or return to an earlier step helps your body stay strong and supported through all stages of motherhood.
2. Integrating core activation into full-body movements like squats and rows builds strength that carries over into everyday mom life.

Unless you've skipped directly to this chapter, you know by now that core training is the foundation of my Core, Function and Fitness approach to mom fitness. Whether pregnant, postpartum, or beyond, core training is essential. I believe that most of you know this; however, the challenge is selecting core exercises that are right for YOU. This chapter will give you the tools to confidently answer those questions, help you identify core exercises for your current stage of motherhood and fitness level, and teach you how to progress safely at your own pace. Can you relate to any of these common questions I've been asked by moms?

- "Can I do planks during pregnancy?"
- "When can I start doing ab workouts after a C-section?"

- "What are the safest exercises to do postpartum?"
- "Why does my back hurt during ab exercises?"
- "Can I get rid of my mommy pooch?"

Five-Step Framework

Step	Goal	Sample Exercises
One: Activation	Coordinate breath with deep core activation	Heel slides Pelvic tilts
Two: Stability	Maintain stability in different positions	Bird dog Planks Bridge marches
Three: Anti-Rotation	Resist rotational forces	Side planks Pallof press Farmer carry
Four: Spinal Flexion	Introduce flexion exercises that target the rectus abdominis	Crunches Reverse crunches
Five: Adding Complexity	Increase challenge by adding resistance or limb movements	Planks with leg lifts Resistance band dead bugs

This five-step framework outlines a progressive approach to core training for moms, from foundational breathwork and deep core activation through functional movement, rotation, spinal flexion, and loaded or complex exercises.

Progressive Core Training

This five-step framework is designed to guide you through core training in a structured, effective way. You'll start at Step One and progress forward, but the journey won't be the same for everyone. Some steps may come easily, while others take more time, or may not be necessary for you at all. As you move through each step, approach it with a personal lens, adapting the progression to fit your unique needs and goals.

Step One: Deep Abdominal Muscle Activation with Breath

The goal of Step One is to master your ability to use breath to connect with your deep core muscles, especially the transverse abdominis (your body's natural "corset"). Activating these muscles with controlled breathing sets the foundation for everything that follows. Whether you're pregnant, early postpartum, or taking your first steps toward fitness years after having a baby, this is where your core training program should begin. As your core training progresses and movements become more advanced, core synergy remains important and ideally will become something that you don't have to think about. For this reason, this stage is foundational regardless of your fitness level or what stage of motherhood you're in.

What Should You Focus On?

Start with simple movements where you don't have to be concerned with form or technique so that you can focus on breathing correctly along with the movement. Your focus should be on whether you feel your TrA activate as you exhale. Some people like to imagine zipping up from the bottom of their pelvis to their ribs or pulling their belly button toward their spine.

Sample Exercises

- **Heel Slides (back):** Lie on your back with your knees bent and feet flat on the floor, hip-width apart. Slowly slide one heel out as you exhale, keeping your abdominal muscles engaged. Pause to inhale (letting your abdominal muscles relax), then reengage your abs, sliding the heel back to the starting position as you exhale. Alternate legs and aim for ten repetitions on each leg.

- **Quadruped Arm Reach:** Start on your hands and knees, with your wrists aligned with your shoulders and knees aligned with your hips. Begin with equal weight distribution from front to back and side to side so that you feel centered, and your hips are level. As you exhale, extend one arm forward without shifting your body. You should be able to feel your abs engage and draw in against gravity. The progression would be to extend the opposite leg as you're extending your arm, keeping your spine neutral and hips level.

- **Standing Single-Arm Dumbbell Front Raise with Core Activation:** Stand with your feet hip-width apart, holding a 3–8-pound dumbbell in one hand with your palm facing your body. As you exhale, keeping your arm straight and wrist neutral, slowly lift your arm forward to shoulder height. Aim to maintain a stable torso without shifting your weight side to side or leaning backward. Pause at the top, then lower your arm back to the starting position with control, letting your abdominal muscles relax as you inhale. Perform five to ten repetitions on each side. Do not work until shoulder fatigue as this is meant to be primarily a core exercise.

Common Mistakes to Avoid

Based on my experience working with moms and moms-to-be, here are some common mistakes.

- "Sucking in" your stomach. The activation and pulling toward your belly button should occur when you exhale, not inhale.
- Assuming you're too advanced for this step. As you improve, you'll notice that you'll "feel" your abs activate immediately even during the most basic exercises. Until activation on the exhale is almost automatic, and you can feel a strong activation no matter the exercise, this step is not too advanced for you.
- Limiting yourself to deep core exercises on your back. Working in multiple positions builds strength and stability that translates into everyday movements, like pulling a stroller out of the trunk or carrying several bags of groceries up the stairs. Once you're comfortable engaging your core on your back, start testing yourself against gravity by standing or performing quadruped exercises.

Considerations for the First through Fourth Trimesters

As your body changes during pregnancy, strengthening your deep core muscles becomes essential for stability and support. Learning how to coordinate breathing and core engagement will help you avoid compensating with other muscles to achieve stability and will help you manage IAP. During the first trimester, you may still feel comfortable performing exercises on your back. In your second and third trimesters, it's generally advised to avoid staying in a supine (lying on your back) position for long periods. As your uterus grows, its weight can press on major blood vessels, potentially reducing blood flow and sometimes making you feel faint. If you start to feel lightheaded, shifting to your left side is a good way to relieve that pressure.

You'll notice I said "long periods" and this is because recent research indicates that while there are some concerns, such as occasional small changes in fetal heart rate during supine exercise, there isn't strong evidence showing that short-term or low-intensity supine exercises (exercises done lying on your back) are harmful to your baby.[1] This is why updated guidelines are less strict than past recommendations that completely advised against back exercises during pregnancy.

If you're within your fourth trimester, it's important to know that there is evidence that your transverse abdominis, one of your key core stabilizers, may not fully regain its contractile strength for up to four months postpartum. This means your core isn't ready for demanding exercises (even if you were consistent in core training during pregnancy), and rushing the process could overload your abdominal and pelvic tissues. It's not uncommon after having a baby, whether C-section or vaginal delivery, for moms to say their abs feel like "mush" or to not be able to feel them activate at all. I'm sharing this to help you manage your expectations and assist in prioritizing where to put your initial effort. Lastly, if you've recently had a baby, most moms can begin breathwork and gentle activation before your postpartum visit as long as it doesn't increase pain or bleeding. Start with simple activities like diaphragmatic breathing or pelvic tilts.

Step Two: Core Stability during Functional Movements

In Step Two, you're building core stability and learning to maintain control as your body moves through more dynamic exercises. Your deep core muscles, including the transverse abdominis, stabilize your spine and pelvis while your arms and legs move independently.

This trains your core to function as a strong, supportive foundation for everyday activities and more complex exercises. The focus is on managing pressure in your core and avoiding movement habits that your body might use to compensate as exercises get more challenging.

What Should You Focus On?

Start by moving beyond core isolation exercises and aiming to activate your core during movements like lunges, squats, and push-ups. These movements train your core to work as part of a team, coordinating with your hips, glutes, and upper body for stability and strength. Focus on maintaining good form, controlled breathing, and deep core engagement rather than just powering through the movement.

Sample Exercises

- **Push-Ups:** Start in a high plank position with your hands under your shoulders and body in a straight line. Inhale as you lower toward the floor, maintaining light core activation against gravity to prevent sinking in your lower back and to keep your torso rigid. Exhale as you press back up, engaging your pelvic floor and deep core muscles right before you begin to return to the start position. For less demand, try push-ups from your knees, a bench, or a wall. Move with control and repeat for three to ten repetitions.

- **Bench-Supported Dumbbell Row:** Place one knee and hand on a bench for support, with your opposite foot on the floor and a dumbbell in your free hand. As you would in a quadruped (hands and knees) position on the floor, ensure proper alignment on the bench with your hip over your knee and shoulder over your wrist. Inhale as you lower the dumbbell toward the floor, resisting the urge to rotate. Exhale as you pull the dumbbell toward your ribs, engaging your pelvic floor and deep stabilizers, similar to a bird dog, to prevent shifting. Move with control and repeat for eight to twelve repetitions on each side.

Common Mistakes to Avoid

Here are some of the mistakes I've seen when integrating core training into functional strength movements:

- Using too little or too much resistance. As you practice engaging your TrA for stability during major movement patterns in everyday life and workouts, you want the movement to be demanding enough that you feel the need to stabilize and can feel your muscles kick in, but you don't want to use too much resistance to where you begin to compensate with other muscles or your form suffers. For example, some of you will feel your core activate during a wall push-up, but others will need a version where gravity adds a greater challenge, like incline push-ups on a bench.

- Losing alignment. Overarching your lower back, tucking your pelvis excessively, or letting your ribs flare can indicate a loss of core control during squats, lunges, deadlifts, push-ups, and pulling exercises. Aim for steady engagement throughout the movement.

- Rushing through reps. Focus on slow, intentional movement until your core starts to kick in automatically before movements that need stability.

Considerations for the First through Fourth Trimesters

Incorporating pelvic floor strengthening during functional movements is beneficial, but as a reminder, if you have hypertonic pelvic floor muscles, your focus should be on fully relaxing your pelvic floor instead. Additionally, whether pregnant or postpartum, if adding resistance to challenge stability increases symptoms of incontinence or pelvic pressure, regress the movement or reduce the weight.

Step Three: Rotation, Anti-Rotation, and Lateral Stability

In this step, you'll challenge your core to resist rotational forces and improve lateral stability, key for balance and control. These exercises target the obliques, deep stabilizers, and the muscles that keep your spine and pelvis aligned when handling uneven loads. Training your body to stay steady against external forces, like a toddler tugging on your arm, carrying an infant car seat in one hand, or controlling twisting movements, helps protect your spine, reduces injury risk, and builds strength for the physical demands of daily life.

What Should You Focus On?

As with the other steps, you'll continue to stay aware of whether your TrA is activating, but it may be harder to feel and intentionally engage other key muscles, like your spinal muscles and obliques. Still, because these muscles are designed to work together, consistently applying the principles from Steps One and Two helps make sure even the muscles you don't feel as easily are doing their job.

Sample Exercises

- **Side Planks:** Lie on your side with your elbow directly under your shoulder and legs stacked or staggered for balance (on your toes or knees). Engage your core and exhale as you lift your hips. Maintain a straight line with your torso, keeping your ribs aligned with your pelvis, and avoid letting your hips sag or rotate forward. Breathe steadily.

- **Pallof Press:** Attach a resistance band or cable at chest height and stand perpendicular to the anchor point, feet hip-width apart. Hold the handle or band at the center of your chest, inhale to prepare, and exhale as you press your hands straight forward, resisting the urge to rotate by engaging your core muscles. Inhale as you bring your hands back to your chest with control and relax your core muscles. Perform eight to twelve repetitions per side.

- **Seated Twists:** Sit with your knees bent and heels flat on the floor. Hold a dumbbell or keep your hands together at your chest. Keep your spine lengthened as you lean back slightly. Inhale as you rotate to one side. Remember to lead with your torso and not your arms. Exhale and engage your core muscles to support you, bringing the weight or hands back to the center starting position. Perform six to twelve repetitions per side.

Common Mistakes to Avoid

Many moms aren't as familiar with proper technique during these types of exercises, so self-assess whether you're making these mistakes:

- Leading with your arms instead of rotating through your torso. Rotational movements should start from your core, not just your arms.

- Over-rotating or twisting through your lower back. Keep your pelvis stable and rotate primarily through your mid-back during rotational exercises. If you have limited mobility in your spine, your range of rotation will be less, so don't force it.

- Relying on momentum instead of controlled movement. Swinging or jerking takes the focus off your core muscles. Move with intention and control, continuing to ensure your breathing coordinates with the movement. Be mindful that your lower body isn't shifting side to side as you twist.

- Losing alignment in standing exercises. In moves like single-arm carries or lateral band walks, keep your shoulders level and avoid leaning toward or away from the weight. Additionally, if walking in a side shuffle, keep your toes pointing forward and avoid your foot turning out toward the side.

Considerations for the First through Fourth Trimesters

While the science on the best way to train obliques during pregnancy and postpartum is limited, we can make reasonable assumptions about rotational exercises and their impact on core function. In general, training your obliques is beneficial, especially when it comes to resisting rotation. However, the type and amount of twisting exercises you perform are where I'd love to see more research.

During pregnancy and postpartum, it's helpful to focus on exercises that train the core to resist rotation (movements like the Pallof press, side-lying hip lifts, and farmer's carries) since they improve stability for everyday tasks. Before adding in rotation, it's important to first ensure that your deep core muscles are activating properly so that the obliques aren't compensating. Since the linea alba naturally stretches during pregnancy and is healing postpartum, excessive twisting or over-recruitment of the obliques could create an additional pull on that tissue. Many moms also experience reduced mid-back mobility during and after pregnancy, making it harder to rotate effectively.

Instead of forcing through that restriction during strength exercises, gentle mobility exercises can help improve movement without adding unnecessary stress to the core.

So, although you may come across general advice to avoid twisting exercises during pregnancy, and while it's true that certain movements should be approached with caution, that doesn't mean oblique training should be ignored altogether.

Step Four: Spinal Flexion

Step Four introduces exercises that engage the rectus abdominis, the superficial "six-pack" muscles, through spinal flexion movements. These exercises involve bending or curling your spine, as in crunches. Because spinal flexion places increased demand on the core, this step typically comes later in the progression framework and is often avoided during the second through fourth trimesters. If your deep core muscles aren't functioning optimally, these exercises can lead to improper muscle activation where the neck, lower back, or hip flexors take over instead of the abdominals. Mastering the foundational core engagement techniques from earlier steps ensures that spinal flexion exercises are performed without compromise.

What Should You Focus On?

By this stage, you should feel confident in your ability to engage your transverse abdominis and coordinate your breath with movement. However, spinal flexion exercises require special attention to ensure the effort stays in your abdominals rather than shifting into your neck or hip flexors. During these more complex exercises that require spinal mobility, focus on continuing to initiate the exercises from your deep core muscles.

Sample Exercises

- **Crunches:** Lie on your back with your knees bent and feet flat on the floor. Place your hands behind your head for light support or across your chest for a less demanding version. Exhale as you engage your core and then lift your head, neck, and shoulders off the ground. Inhale as you lower back down with control.
- **V-Ups:** Lie on your back with your legs extended and arms overhead. Engage your core and exhale as you lift your legs and upper body at the same time, reaching your hands toward your toes. Lower back down with control, not letting your pelvis tilt as your legs get closer to the ground.

Common Mistakes to Avoid

Despite flexion exercises being the most commonly performed ab exercises, this is often where I see big mistakes. Try to avoid the following:

- Pulling on your neck. If your hands are behind your head, keep your elbows wide and lightly support your head with your fingertips. Aim for a neutral neck position with a slight space between your chin and chest, as if holding an apple under your chin.
- Not controlling the lowering phase (eccentric contraction). To fully engage the core, lower your upper body with control down to the floor. We know that in other areas of the body, eccentric exercises are known to improve muscle strength, size, and structure more than other types of muscle actions, so the same may apply to the rectus abdominis as well.

- Pushing through too many repetitions. Quality matters more than quantity. Fatigue often leads to compensations like using momentum, straining the neck, or losing core engagement. If form breaks down, it's better to stop or modify the movement rather than push through.

Considerations for the First through Fourth Trimesters

Most moms-to-be stop doing spinal flexion exercises after the first trimester, not just because a growing bump makes them more awkward but also because they increase intra-abdominal pressure without offering much benefit at that stage. While spinal mobility in all directions still matters, core strengthening through flexion isn't essential during pregnancy since the rectus abdominis is already stretching to make room for your baby and isn't a key stabilizer.

The same logic applies postpartum. Early on, focusing on Steps One, Two, and Three will better support the demands of motherhood than jumping into spinal flexion. Once you're confident in your deep core engagement and your abdominal tissues have had time to heal and regain strength, you can gradually reintroduce those exercises. As a side note, growing evidence suggests that exercises like crunches and other spinal flexion movements do not increase the risk of diastasis recti or delay healing in postpartum moms, and in some cases, they may even be beneficial.[2] So, progressing to this step is important for all moms.

Step Five: Adding Resistance and Complexity

By Step Five, your core should be strong enough to handle greater challenges. Adding resistance through bands, dumbbells, and cables, or adding complexity to the exercises you're already doing, proves invaluable for overloading your muscles, so you can keep progressing.

As a mom, your core is constantly under load from daily activities like lifting, carrying, and bending, so building strength and stability with added resistance prepares you for both the demands of motherhood and your personal fitness goals. Depending on where you begin your prenatal core progression, some expecting moms will also find it useful to use resistance or add complexity for continued strength and function.

What Should You Focus On?

As you add resistance or complexity, your goal is to maintain the same abdominal stability you developed in earlier steps. This step elevates your training toward muscular development while reinforcing the dynamic support and coordinated movement patterns you've already established.

Sample Exercises

- **Dead Bugs with Resistance Bands:** Holding a band attached to a stable anchor further challenges your core by forcing your muscles to resist being pulled out of position

- **Pallof Press Variations:** Use heavier resistance or vary the movement by pressing overhead or changing positions like performing it from a kneeling position or a different angle.

- **Lunges with Rotation:** If you've been holding a dumbbell during lunges, try adding a rotation to challenge stability. As you step forward into the lunge, rotate your torso toward the front leg, keeping the movement controlled and initiated from your core rather than your arms. Return to the center as you push back to standing.

- **Planks:** From a knee or full plank position, extend one arm out to the side and lightly tap the floor, then return to the starting position. Alternate arms while keeping your hips steady and core engaged to resist rotation.

Common Mistakes to Avoid

- Holding your breath. With added resistance, you may feel the need to brace your core more than in other steps. This can be a helpful stabilizing technique as what's called the Valsalva Maneuver increases IAP, especially when it comes to heavy lifting.[3] However, remember that increased IAP could impact your pelvic floor muscles.

- Jumping ahead. You may be ready for more complex exercises or adding resistance, but just as you've done to get to this point, adding challenge requires progression. In future chapters, we'll talk about progressive overload, which by definition is a "gradual" increase of stress placed on your muscles over time. This step is no exception. If you're increasing the weight of your dumbbells, do so incrementally, allowing your body a chance to adapt before adding more weight. If you're adding a side arm tap with the planks, consider trying it from your knees before returning to full planks.

Considerations for the First through Fourth Trimesters

If you're pregnant and progressing to Step Five, make sure you're weighing the benefits of added resistance and complexity. Adding dumbbells or advancing an exercise will most likely increase IAP and depending on where you are in your pregnancy and how your body is responding to your growing baby, you may choose to skip this step and maintain what you've been doing or progress through this step at a more gradual pace.

Step Five is a huge milestone for postpartum moms. It means you've been consistent, allowed your body time to heal, have a core that's functioning as it should, have built basic strength, and your emphasis can shift to muscle definition and increased strength. If you've made it to this step, I encourage you to celebrate and reassess your fitness goals, as it most likely means you can take on more vigorous physical activity. But still, remember that even if you're ready to add complexity or resistance, you should do it progressively.

How Do You Know When to Progress to the Next Step?

Remember that any forward progress is progress, and the pace at which you move through each step will vary based on your individual situation and will be unique to your needs, effort, and consistency. Your ability to assess and follow the framework will guide your advancement, but here are some general indicators you're ready for the next phase:

- You can perform two to three sets of eight to fifteen repetitions, maintaining proper breath control and deep core engagement.
- You can feel the right muscles firing at the right time. For example, if you can perform a push-up but your lower back lags, the right muscles aren't yet working when they need to.
- You're bored or have plateaued. If you've been performing the same routine consistently for longer than eight to twelve weeks, it's probably time to mix things up.
- You can maintain technique and form even when fatigued.

- You can complete the exercise through a full range of motion comfortably and without tightness or restriction limiting your movement.

When Should You Return to Previous Steps or Regress an Exercise?

Most of the time, your core training program will focus on progressing by adding more muscles, movements, and resistance. However, during certain stages of motherhood, like during pregnancy or postpartum recovery, you should be open to regressing. Here are some key situations when taking a step back can support your long-term strength and function:

- As you move from trimester to trimester, spinal flexion exercises and targeted rectus abdominis work become less of a priority, and regressing is a good idea when the benefits no longer outweigh the risks.
- If you've recently had a baby, even if you maintained strength and progressed exercises during pregnancy, your priority should be rebuilding your core foundation, which means returning to Step One.
- If you experience pain or discomfort, regression may help address symptoms related to overuse, overtraining, an injury, or a pelvic health condition. Returning to a previous step may help you rebuild foundational strength and function.
- When adding weight or resistance, regressing the movement pattern may be necessary to master the technique under the new challenge. For example, if you've progressed to a wide-

stance bridge march but decide to add a weight plate to your hips, you may need to narrow your foot position until you adjust to the increased load.

Are There Times When You Should Skip a Step?

Yes. While progression is the goal, there are certain situations where skipping a step or portion of a step may be the best approach. Here are a few scenarios when modifying your path forward makes sense:

- If rotational exercises cause SI joint pain, low back discomfort, or aggravate your round ligament, you can skip the rotational exercises in Step Three. Instead, focus on targeting the same muscle groups through anti-rotation exercises.

- During pregnancy, spinal flexion exercises like crunches, hollow holds, and full dead bugs are generally not recommended once your belly begins to show. Instead, skipping this step and continuing to Step Five and finding additional ways to challenge your core make sense.

Skipping a step does not mean skipping progress. It's about making informed choices based on your body's needs and ensuring that each movement serves your long-term strength and function. I'll continue to say it . . . exercise is a tool.

Time to Put the Framework to Practical Use

This core training framework isn't meant to be rigid. It's designed to empower you to start and stay active in a way that's both effective and adaptable. Over the years, this approach has helped hundreds of moms regain strength and confidence, and it can do the same for you.

With this information you should be able to evaluate whether you're in the right fitness class. If a class is focused on advanced movements like planks with leg lifts or weighted exercises (Step Five), but you haven't yet built foundational strength in Step One, it may not be the best fit for you yet. Beyond the physical readiness factor, being in a class that feels too advanced can be emotionally discouraging, especially as a busy, sleep-deprived mom.

Take Andrea, a mom I worked with after she had twins. Although holding a plank wasn't her primary goal, progressing through her core training and eventually achieving her first-ever plank became a huge source of pride. It was a reminder of how strong her body was, not just in carrying twins but also in recovering and growing stronger postpartum. If she had joined a class where she struggled to keep up, she might have felt discouraged and deprioritizing exercise altogether. The right program can make all the difference in how you feel about your body, and this framework helps ensure you're in the right place. And as a fun side note, her sister started training with me, too, and ended up doing her first push-up ever! A coincidence? I think not!

Another use for this framework is to determine your starting point. If you haven't exercised consistently for a while, begin with Step One to build core awareness and stability before adding complexity.

Lastly, these five steps will help you recognize when you're ready to progress or when it makes sense to regress. This approach to core training gives you a clear path forward while also helping you identify when stepping back is the smartest move for long-term strength and success. By using this approach, you'll master the Core portion of CFF, creating a foundation that you can build from for a lifetime.

If You Want Variety

If you enjoy switching up your workouts or want to challenge your core in new ways, incorporating different tools can add variety. Here are some of my favorites:

- Suspension trainers: Suspension training makes traditional core exercises more challenging by increasing instability. In Step Five, try advanced plank variations or pike progressions to build strength while improving coordination and balance.
- BOSU: Adding instability to exercises like planks, mountain climbers, and push-ups forces deeper core engagement. I also love using it for crunch variations, as it helps stabilize the pelvis and prevent unnecessary strain. This is a great tool for Steps Two, Three, Four, and Five.
- Foam roller: This can be a useful addition for both core strength and mobility. Unstable holds and rolling plank variations enhance activation, while the roller also helps release tight back and hip flexor muscles, common areas of tension for moms. You can use this tool as early as Step One, especially if restriction in your back impacts your breathing.
- Sliding discs/gliders: These introduce a fun yet challenging way to add dynamic movement to your core workouts. Try mountain climbers or planks with controlled arm or leg slides. Introducing gliders into Step One can even make heel slides more fun.
- Pilates ball (9-inch mini ball): I've had the most success teaching moms how to activate their TrA with this simple piece of equipment. By placing it behind your lower back during seated exercises or under your ribs in side-lying movements,

you'll receive tactile feedback to keep your pelvis stable. This is useful in the early steps, but you'll also feel a nice burn using the ball in Steps Four and Five in exercises like crunches.

Back to the Common Questions

Now that we're approaching the end of this chapter, you may know the answers to some questions, but let's revisit them together with some added clarity.

"Why does my back/neck hurt during ab exercises?"

Discomfort is often a sign that your body is compensating. When your deep core muscles aren't activating effectively, your hip flexors, neck, or lower back may take over. If this sounds familiar, it's a sign that you may need to revisit Step One to improve your connection to the deep core. Focus on breathwork and engagement before increasing difficulty.

"When can I start doing ab workouts after a C-section?"

The first step in rebuilding core strength isn't crunches or planks, it's breathwork. As soon as you feel up to it, you can begin reconnecting with your transverse abdominis and pelvic floor through gentle breathing and muscle activation exercises. Before progressing to more dynamic exercises, check with your doctor to ensure your incision is healing well and that you have a plan for scar tissue management.

One thing I've noticed from working with moms is that C-section recovery doesn't always feel linear. The first four to eight weeks can be taxing, and then suddenly, you wake up one day feeling significantly better. I don't share this to set expectations but to reassure you that if progress feels slow at first, don't get demoralized. You will regain strength and movement; it just might happen in unexpected leaps rather than a steady climb.

"Should I do planks?"

Typically, this question is asked during pregnancy or postpartum, but hopefully, you've learned that no matter what stage of motherhood you're in, the decision should be based on whether you can engage your core muscles effectively against gravity, without holding your breath. Until we have more research, the "safety" of planks during pregnancy will probably remain a gray area. If you're comfortable with them and can maintain good form, go for it. If they don't feel right, and you're content doing alternative exercises to maintain core strength and function during pregnancy, then skip them.

"Can I get rid of my mommy pooch?"

This is one of the hardest questions to answer because it's tied to emotion, societal pressure, and adjusting to a new body. The truth is that several factors influence how your stomach looks postpartum. If your skin was stretched significantly during pregnancy, it will take a combination of hydration, healing, nutrition, and exercise to see changes. If you have DRA, it may impact the appearance of your stomach. If you had a C-section, you may notice a "shelf" around the incision, which can take time to soften and change. Some moms notice that their body holds on to extra fat while breastfeeding. Genetics, hormones, stress, sleep, and age all play a role in body composition and how your core responds postpartum. The appearance of your stomach is a reflection of body composition, the balance of muscle, fat, and skin. Because so many factors influence your fat-to-muscle ratio and the elasticity of your skin, I encourage you to instead concentrate on strength and function alongside hydration and nutrition. While no one can predict exactly how your stomach will look, with consistency, you will see progress and feel stronger.

Final Thoughts

I hope this chapter has given you confidence that a strong and functional core is possible, no matter where you're starting from. Learning how to train effectively and progressively not only helps you feel and move better but also gives you the power to be stronger than you were before pregnancy. Core training is just one, but a very important, piece of the CFF pie chart.

Take Action

If you're ready to apply what you've learned, choose from these next steps (see Appendix B for more resources on progressive core training):

1. Review Steps One through Five and pick the one that feels right based on your current fitness level, stage of motherhood, symptoms, or confidence. Start with one recommended exercise from that step and practice it with focused breath and form.

2. Look at your current exercise routine or favorite fitness class. Are you doing planks, crunches, or loaded movements without a foundation? If so, use the framework to identify whether you might benefit from stepping back to strengthen your base.

Part III

7

Master These (Mom) Movements

> **Key Insights from This Chapter**
> - Common movements like pushing, pulling, hinging, lunging, rotating, and squatting directly link to your daily actions and are strengthened through targeted functional training.
> - Ensuring major muscles fire at the right time and work in collaboration with supporting muscles improves your training efficiency and helps you avoid compensation and pain.

It's a Saturday morning and you're six months pregnant with your second child. Your alarm clock, also known as your two-year-old, is yelling your name from the other room. You slowly roll out of bed and make your way down the hall to start your day. Fortunately, he's beyond the stage of climbing out of his crib, so he's standing there with his arms outstretched just waiting for you. After you lift him out of the crib, you place him on your hip, reach back in for his favorite stuffy, and then carry him to the bathroom to be changed. Next up, it's time for breakfast, so you grab his hand, gripping it lightly as you both walk down the stairs. At the bottom of the stairs, you notice the basket of laundry you forgot to put in the washer last night. After lifting your child into the booster seat and giving him a cup of water, you head back to the stairs, grab the basket, and rush back upstairs to start a load of whites. You're on your way back down the hallway to go make breakfast, when you notice a few toys on the floor, so you bend down, pick them up, and toss them in your child's room, making it back down the stairs just in time for your child to say, "mommy I'm hungry."

You managed to get yourself and your child fed, glance at the clock, and realize you still have hours before he naps. You decide to take advantage of a beautiful day and go have some fun at the park. You take your son's hand in your right hand and put your left hand on your belly, wondering if your unborn daughter will enjoy the park just like your son. Your son quickly brings you out of your daydream when he takes off running down the sidewalk. He's fast, but you were able to react quickly and grab his shoulder to stop him. You return to the house to get the diaper bag and grab the stroller out of the trunk. You've become a master at one-handed activities because you don't want to let go of his hand before he's safely buckled in the stroller. It's your lucky day, and he doesn't put up a fight, so after securing your water bottle in the cup holder, you're on your way.

After ten minutes of pushing him on the swings, he's gathered up some courage and is trying to climb with the big kids. He climbs higher on the ladder than ever before, making both of you proud, but he hasn't yet mastered getting down safely. You reach up and put your hands on his waist to assist him back to the ground. Satisfied with the outing, you decide it's time to head home for lunch. Your son disagrees, and you struggle to get him in the stroller. Feeling the exhaustion of pregnancy, you pick your battles and let him walk beside you instead. You hold his hand in your left, as you guide the stroller with your right. Back at home, you both eat a quick lunch, he goes down for a nap easily, and you sit down on the couch wondering if you should curl up and also take a nap or if you should get up to put the clothes in the dryer.

Whether you're pregnant and don't have any other children or are a mom of three, we all can relate to the tasks, thoughts, and feelings occurring in this routine. I'd ask that now you also consider all of the familiar actions in this routine and the strength, energy, balance, and coordination required. Going up and down the stairs, lifting, walking, carrying, and dashing might seem like ordinary moments, but they highlight just how physically demanding motherhood is.

My Core, Function, and Fitness approach to maternal exercise prioritizes functional strength training to prepare you for the real-life demands of motherhood in addition to fitness. By focusing on movement patterns like pushing, pulling, and hinging, you train your muscles to work together so that you can perform daily tasks efficiently and comfortably. In the previous chapter, you learned about the foundation of CFF, and now it's time to move to the next layer of the pyramid or shift the proportions of your pie chart and focus on function. Keep in mind that your core plays an essential role in functional strength training, so you'll continue to apply the principles from Chapter 6. It's time to move through your day with ease and your workouts with strength and confidence!

Mom Movement Chart

The following chart is a quick summary showing you how common actions directly connect to movement patterns that can be improved by functional strength training. Each movement pattern is supported by ensuring the major muscles involved are strong and that they coordinate with the secondary muscles involved in the movement.

Just as we discussed with your core, to perform these movements or exercises without pain or compensation, and to build lasting strength and function, the right muscles have to engage at the right time.

Movement Pattern	Mom Movement	Sample Exercises
Push	Pushing a stroller or heavy door	Wall push-up or dumbbell chest press
Pull	Sliding a car seat toward you to pull out of the car or helping your child up from the floor	TRX row or seated cable row
Squat	Sitting on a chair or picking up a laundry hamper	Body weight squat or goblet squat
Lunge	Kneeling to buckle a stroller or crouching to reach a low shelf at the store	Reverse lunge or walking lunge
Hinge	Lifting your child out of the crib or picking them up from the floor	Deadlift or glute bridge
Rotation/anti-rotation	Reaching into the backseat or carrying a child on one hip	Reverse lunge or walking lunge

This chart identifies six fundamental movement patterns regularly performed in motherhood (push, pull, squat, lunge, hinge, and rotation/anti-rotation) and provides examples of real-life "mom movements" to connect everyday tasks with functional fitness strategies.

How to Train Movement Patterns

In this section, I'll break down the key movement patterns you should master with helpful tips and mistakes to avoid based on my experience coaching hundreds of moms. It's now time to shift your perspective and read with your personal needs and goals in mind. It's not a bad idea as you start to decipher what the following information means to you, to go back to the personal assessment you took earlier in the book, as well as ensure that you've identified where you are in the core training framework. Let's dive into the middle layer of CFF!

Mom Movement: Pushing

The primary muscles involved in pushing are the chest, shoulders, and back of your arms, also known as pectoralis major, deltoids (primarily the anterior deltoid), and triceps brachii. The push pattern shows up in your daily life in actions like pushing a swing, stroller, or heavy door. These actions may seem simple, but not only do they require muscle strength, but coordinating the movement with core activation is also an essential skill to learn.

Sample Push Pattern Exercises

- Push-up variations: Stability ball wall push-ups, full body with hands narrow, or feet elevated with an eccentric focus.
- Shoulder press variations: Seated presses with dumbbells and palms facing each other, standing presses with a barbell overhand grip, cable machine presses at an angle.

Tips

- Exhale and engage your core right before performing the push part of the exercise.
- Hold strong in your upper back and shoulder area. Don't let your shoulder blades collapse inward toward each other.

Common Push-Up Mistakes to Avoid

- Not trying to do push-ups because you've never been successful. Core engagement plays a huge role, and with a strong core foundation, you will find a push-up variation that you're able to do.

- Thinking that knee push-ups are the only way to practice and progress to full push-ups. If you're unable to do full push-ups, it could be due to primary muscle weakness, but it could also be that you lack shoulder stability or have restricted upper-body mobility. To improve at push-ups, you may need to address these issues separately with exercises like wall angels or band pulls.

- Reaching with your head or neck rather than lowering your torso to get to the bottom phase of the push-up. During push-ups, your body should move and lower as a unit.

Prenatal/Postpartum Consideration

Remember that exercises like push-ups force your core to work against gravity, which requires more IAP. This does not mean you should avoid these exercises, but you should be mindful of the amount of IAP required and make sure you're gradually progressing to more advanced versions of these exercises.

Mom Movement: Pulling

The primary muscles involved in pulling are the upper back, shoulders, and front of your arms, also known as the latissimus dorsi, trapezius, rhomboids, posterior deltoid, and biceps brachii. The pull pattern shows up in your daily life in actions like sliding a car seat out of the car, helping your child up from the floor, or attempting to maintain upper-body posture. These movements may seem simple, but they require not just upper-body strength but also coordination with your core to stabilize and support the motion effectively.

Sample Pull Pattern Exercises

- Row variations: seated cable rows, hinged dumbbell rows, or single-arm bench rows
- Lat pulldowns: overhand grip with resistance bands, underhand grip on a cable machine
- Pull-ups: overhand grip on a bar, narrow grip palms facing each other, underhand grip on a suspension trainer

Tips

- Exhale throughout the entire pull and inhale as you control the release.
- Envision the muscles around your shoulder blades activating just before you start to bend at your elbows and engage your arm muscles.

Common Pull-Up or Rowing Mistakes to Avoid

- Shrugging your shoulders toward your ears instead of keeping them down and engaging your upper back for stability.
- Pulling with just your arms rather than initiating the movement from your back muscles.

Prenatal/Postpartum Consideration

Rowing is an effective exercise to combat the forward pull caused by the weight of your belly or breasts. However, similar to push-ups, hinged rows without bench support require you to work against gravity and demand more core engagement than a seated cable row, for example. If you're concerned about the ability to engage your core, select exercises with less demand on your deep core muscles.

Mom Movement: Squatting

The primary muscles involved in squatting are the front and back of your thighs, and your glutes, also known as the quadriceps, gluteus maximus, and hamstrings. These muscles work together to help you lower and lift your body with control, while your core and hips provide stability. The squat pattern shows up in your daily life in actions like sitting down and standing up, lifting your child from the floor, or bending to load and unload the dishwasher. These movements may seem simple, but they require not just lower body strength but also coordination with your core to maintain balance, protect your back, and move efficiently.

Sample Squat Pattern Exercises

- Squat variations: goblet squats, wall squats, or plié squats
- Weighted squats: holding dumbbells, Smith machine back squats, or barbell front squats
- Balance-focused squats: on a BOSU, single-leg squats

Tips

- As you rise from the squat, press through your heels to activate your glutes so that squats aren't always quad-dominant.
- To improve the range of motion of your squats, ensure adequate ankle and hip mobility.
- Inhale as you lower into the squat and exhale as you return to a standing position, engaging your core especially if performing weighted squats.

Common Squatting Mistakes to Avoid

- Allowing your knees to collapse inward.
- Shifting your weight onto your toes instead of keeping it evenly distributed or centered in your heels.
- Leaning too far forward, turning the movement into a hinge instead of a squat.

Prenatal/Postpartum Consideration

As your center of gravity shifts, exercises like squats may feel different than they used to. Adjusting your base of support (foot positioning) can help you find more stability and balance. Try a wider stance, turning your toes slightly outward or placing a resistance band above your knees to cue your glutes. If ankle stiffness from swelling or prolonged inactivity is limiting your range of motion, slightly elevating your heels on a small weight plate or dumbbell can help you achieve better squat depth without compromising core engagement.

Mom Movement: Lunging

The primary muscles involved in squatting are the front and back of your thighs, and your glutes, also known as the quadriceps, gluteus maximus, and hamstrings. Your core and smaller hip stabilizers help you maintain balance and control throughout the movement. The lunge pattern shows up in your daily life in actions like stepping forward to clean up toys, kneeling to buckle a stroller, or crouching to reach a low shelf at the store. These movements may seem simple, but they require not just lower body strength but also single-leg stability, core engagement, and control to stay balanced in an asymmetrical stance or when shifting your weight from one leg to the other.

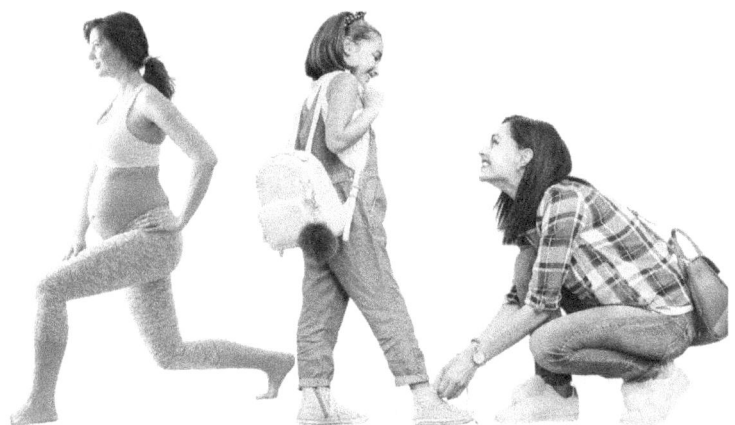

Real-life and exercise examples of the lunge pattern. **Left:** *A mom performing a stationary lunge, highlighting the lunge movement pattern in exercise.* Zukovic via Getty Images. **Right:** *A mom tying her child's shoe, highlighting the lunge movement pattern in everyday life.* martin-dm via Getty Images.

Sample Lunge Pattern Exercises

- Straight-line lunges: forward, reverse, see saw, stationary with support, deficit
- Multidirectional lunges: lateral, curtsy, clock
- Dynamic or advanced lunges: walking, Bulgarian split squats, jump lunges

Tips

- Keep your front knee stacked over your ankle for less force on the knee.
- Inhale as you lower into the lunge and exhale as you return to a standing position.
- Distribute weight through your front heel instead of shifting onto your toes to increase glute engagement.

Common Lunging Mistakes to Avoid

- Pushing off your back leg instead of driving through your front foot and glute.
- Leaning your torso forward or rounding your shoulders, reducing core engagement.
- Dropping your back heel instead of staying on the ball of your foot between repetitions.

Prenatal/Postpartum Consideration

Although lunging is an essential movement pattern for moms, if you're experiencing pain from SPD or other pelvic girdle issues, traditional lunges may aggravate symptoms. To maintain lunging benefits like balance, coordination, and single-leg stability with less strain, try kickstand squats or narrow-stance lunges. If discomfort persists, temporarily avoid lunges and focus on strengthening your glutes, quadriceps, and hamstrings through isolated exercises or squat and hinge variations that feel comfortable.

Mom Movement: Hinging

The primary muscles involved in hinging are the glutes, back of your legs, and lower back, also known as the gluteus maximus, hamstrings, and erector spinae. Your deep core stabilizers and upper back muscles also play a role in maintaining proper posture throughout the movement. The hinge pattern can be done vertically, like in deadlifts, or horizontally, like in hip thrusts or glute bridges. Hinging shows up in your daily life in actions like bending to pick up your child, lifting your baby out of the crib, or reaching down when a deep squat feels uncomfortable during pregnancy. Training this movement strengthens the posterior chain, improves posture, and reduces strain on your lower back.

I have to mention two of the moms I worked with, one during pregnancy and the other postpartum. I can still remember their "aha moments" of mastering the deadlift. It's a tough movement to do because the body instinctively wants to begin the movement like a squat, and it requires primary activation of the glutes and hamstrings, which doesn't come as easily as activation of the quadriceps, for most people. I believe the most helpful cue for both of them ended up being, "Close the car door with your butt," which was the key for them to initiate the movement by pushing their hips back rather than leaning their torso forward. It really can be the little things. If you're a former client reading this and think I'm talking about you, I probably am! And I thank you for allowing us to spend weeks perfecting the move! More importantly, I think this is a testament to the value I place on this exercise for moms at all stages of motherhood. At the Active Mom Fitness studio, it was the exercise that moms were the most inexperienced with, yet the one I wanted them to learn the most because it can absolutely change your quality of life and improve fitness.

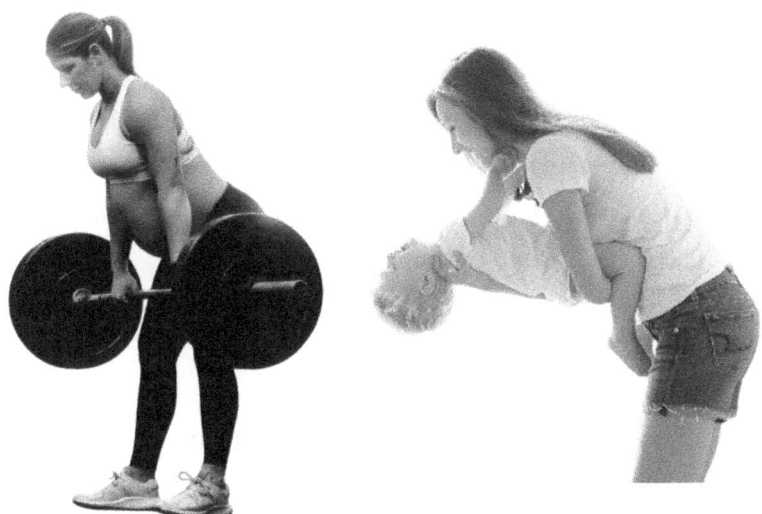

Real-life and exercise examples of the hinge pattern. **Left:** *A mom performing a deadlift, demonstrating how hip hinging is used in both daily tasks and strength training.* RyanJLane via Getty Images. **Right:** *A mom lifting her child from the floor, demonstrating how hip hinging is used in both daily tasks and strength training.* Cavan Images via Getty Images.

Sample Hinge Pattern Exercises

- Deadlift variations: Romanian with a kettlebell, single-leg with a dumbbell on the same side or opposite arm, stiff leg with a barbell

- Hip thrust variations: on a machine, single-leg using a couch, knee-banded
- Glute bridge variations: with a barbell, feet elevated, single-leg with pulses

Tips for Deadlifts

- Begin the exercise by pushing your hips back rather than bending forward at the waist or initiating the exercise by bending at your knees.
- Engage your upper back to prevent your shoulders from being pulled forward and your mid-back from rounding.
- Shift your weight slightly to the outside of your heels to activate your glutes and support your lower back.
- Inhale as your hips hinge and torso lowers, and exhale as you return to a standing position.

Tips for Hip Thrusts and Glute Bridges

- Use a bench or couch at about knee height, so you can rest your upper back comfortably on the edge.
- Keep your feet about hip-width apart and under your knees at the top of the thrust to ensure you're dominating with your glutes and not your quads.
- Shift your weight slightly to the outside of your heels to activate your glutes.
- Inhale as your hips dip and exhale as your hips lift.

Common Deadlift Mistakes to Avoid

- Holding weights too far from your shins during a deadlift increases strain on your back.
- Using your lower back instead of your glutes and hamstrings to lift.
- Rolling your pelvis during a glute bridge (this is okay in hip thrusts but not bridges).

Common Hip Thrust and Glute Bridge Mistakes to Avoid

- Feet too far out, shifting the emphasis to your hamstrings or too close, overemphasizing your quads.
- Letting your head drop back or moving your neck forward and back as your body lifts up and down.
- Not lowering your hips fully during a hip thrust or keeping the glutes contracted without relaxing to reengage the glutes.
- Rolling your pelvis during a glute bridge (rolling slightly is OK in hip thrusts).
- Flaring your ribs or hyperextending your lower back during a bridge.

Prenatal/Postpartum Consideration

Hip hinge exercises are one of the best ways to strengthen your glutes during and after pregnancy; however, for various reasons, one version or another may not work for you. For example, you may choose to avoid glute bridges because you don't want to exercise on your back during the second and third trimesters. Or if you didn't master deadlifts in your first trimester, attempting in your third trimester may feel more difficult due to a lack of upper back strength or tightness in your hamstrings. Things like getting in and out of a hip thrust might become difficult toward the end of your pregnancy or cause discomfort during the fourth trimester. But, because this movement pattern is so valuable, I encourage you to prioritize finding a version that you can perform or determine what the inhibiting factor is, so you troubleshoot how to address it.

Mom Movement: Rotation or Anti-Rotation

The primary muscles involved in anti-rotation and rotational movements are the obliques (internal and external), transverse abdominis, and rectus abdominis. Your glutes (primarily the glute medius) and quadratus lumborum (a deep lower back muscle) also play key roles in maintaining control and stability, but we'll talk about those in the next chapter. Rotation and resisting rotation show up in daily life when carrying a child on one hip, reaching behind you to the back seat to give your baby a pacifier, or grabbing dishes from a dishwasher on your right side and placing them in a high cabinet on your left side. Strengthening these movement patterns enhances your ability to safely twist, reach, and carry asymmetrical loads, without straining your spine.

Sample Rotational and Anti-Rotational Pattern Exercises

- Pallof press variations: press-out horizontally, side shuffle, press up vertically
- Side planks: from your knees, full body, or with an added reach up.

- Woodchops: standing with a resistance band anchored low, kneeling with a cable anchored high, or with a dumbbell.

Tips

- During rotations, picture your waist like a dishrag, ringing the water out.
- Improve mobility with exercises like thread-the-needle or foam rolling if you feel restricted in rotation or pain when resisting rotation.
- When rotating with a band or cable, initiate the movement from your torso, not just your arms.
- During side planks, aim to place more weight on your lower body and align your elbow directly under your shoulder to reduce pressure on the joint.

Common Anti-Rotation Mistakes to Avoid

- Letting your shoulders or hips rotate in anti-rotational movements, rather than using your core to resist rotation.
- Not having the right foot position in standing exercises. Consider a width where you feel steady but still challenged.

Common Rotation Mistakes to Avoid

- Rotating from your lower back (lumbar spine) instead of your mid-back (thoracic spine) or trying to rotate more than the mobility you have in your back allows.
- Not pivoting through your hips in standing rotations. Use your glutes to avoid twisting solely through your spine.

Prenatal/Postpartum Consideration

Many of the considerations for rotational and anti-rotational exercises were covered in the previous chapter, so I'll take this opportunity to emphasize that if you're not ready for rotational exercises, anti-rotation is just as important, if not more, during and after pregnancy. Instead of skipping this movement pattern entirely, focus on mastering exercises that help you resist rotational forces, like your toddler tugging on one hand.

Master the Movements

There was a lot of information in this chapter, and I don't expect you to master all of these movement patterns after just one read or one workout. In fact, "master" is a strong word, especially since each movement pattern has many variations. What I really want you to take away is that to move through daily life without discomfort and to get the most out of your training, you need to develop solid technique and ensure the primary muscles are playing their part during each exercise.

Even with the tips, common mistakes, and considerations, some of you may still struggle with certain movements. This could be because the exercise is too advanced, you have mobility restrictions, your coordination isn't quite there yet, your core needs more foundational strength, or supporting muscles aren't activating as they should. Skipping over these challenges instead of addressing them can cause you to feel stuck or frustrated with exercise. But if you take the time to practice, identify what's holding you back, and adjust, you will build functional strength. In the next chapter, I'll give you even more guidance to help you do just that, so keep reading!

Take Action

If you're ready to put this into practice, choose one of the following next steps:

1. Pay attention to how you move during daily activities like lifting your child, crouching, or pushing a stroller. Consider the movement pattern associated with these activities and reflect on whether it would be beneficial to focus on functional training to make these movements more efficient and comfortable.

2. Review Appendix B for additional resources to support you in mastering these movements!

8

Isolated Muscle Training for Strength and Mobility

> ### *Key Insights from This Chapter*
> - Isolated muscle training strengthens key muscles that support full-body movements, making everyday tasks like lifting, carrying, and getting up from the floor feel more stable and controlled.
> - Pregnancy and postpartum changes can overwork some muscles while others become less active; targeting these muscles directly helps improve strength, posture, and stability.

In the previous chapter, we covered the Function aspect of the CFF model, focusing on the importance of mastering movement patterns. Now, we'll spotlight the supporting muscles that help the primary muscles do their job as you perform those exercises. During pregnancy, anatomical shifts and posture changes can cause certain muscles to tighten or become overactive, while others may need targeted strengthening. After pregnancy, as your body adjusts again, and you take your first steps toward fitness, repetitive postures and movements like feeding your baby and carrying the infant seat create new physical demands. While the CFF approach emphasizes training movement patterns rather than individual muscles (as discussed in the previous chapter), if you find it challenging to perform them, extra attention to an individual muscle or joint could be beneficial.

Common Movement Challenges

I'd like us to start this section by discussing a few common scenarios that you may be able to relate to. If you've experienced any of these, you've probably also experienced negative self-talk, maybe blaming yourself for not "being in shape," feeling guilty for not stretching more, or blaming stress and tension for discomfort. After reading this chapter, I hope that you understand that the frustration you're feeling with your body during these common movement challenges could be tied to very specific muscles not working as they should, rather than something as all-encompassing as you needing to "be more fit" or you being unskilled at an exercise.

Getting Up and Down from the Floor with Baby

Whether you're on the floor for a diaper change or mid-tummy time, there comes a point when you need to stand up, with your baby in your arms. If that moment feels shaky or you're unsure about your balance while holding your little one, you're not alone. What seems like a simple task actually requires coordination of core and hip muscles and single-leg strength. While lunges are an effective way to train your body to go from the floor to standing, you will find stability and control difficult if the muscles that attach to your pelvis lack the required strength and coordination to perform this pattern well. Meaning, to master the lunge, you may need to target your hip stabilizers or rotators.

Upper Back and Neck Pain during Daily Tasks

Whether you spend hours hunched in front of a computer or wear your baby in a front carrier position every day while attempting to get them to nap, forward postures can cause tension or even pain in your neck and upper back. Not only is the soreness aggravating, but the lack of flexibility and strength in your chest and mid-back can impact your ability to deadlift, row, squat, and more. This is another case where targeted training may be necessary to master movement patterns and address discomfort.

Lower Back Pain during Daily Tasks

Whether you're picking up a toy, lifting the car seat, or leaning over the crib, low back pain can turn those tasks into a struggle. But, if I did my job in the previous chapter, you're hopefully eager to incorporate hip hinge exercises into your exercise routine to better protect your spine during these movements. However, if you're finding it difficult to master this movement pattern, targeted training can help you develop the mobility and control needed to perform the hip hinge correctly and move more comfortably throughout your day.

Time to Target Train

From the examples provided, I hope you now understand that if you're unable to perform those movements correctly, additional training for specific muscles can be crucial. Paying attention to these supporting muscles made all the difference for moms like Jamie whose reduced ankle mobility was preventing proper squat form during pregnancy, or moms like Xochi whose increased back mobility enabled years of exercise consistency rather than daily pain, or how Narissa's improved shoulder stability and core strength led to push-up variations she never thought possible. In this next section, we'll address a short list of muscles that frequently need bonus attention, and at the end of the chapter, I'll provide you with example exercises so that instead of feeling frustrated with your body, you feel confident in how you perform the major movement patterns and how you move throughout pregnancy, postpartum, and beyond!

Around the Pelvis

Many of the muscles most affected by pregnancy and postpartum changes connect to the pelvis. As the anchor point for key muscles that support movements like squats, lunges, and hip hinges, the pelvis plays a central role in how your lower body functions. That's why I often refer to this approach as "working our way around the pelvis." It's a way to build workouts in a logical sequence, targeting the muscles that support and stabilize this area. Whether pregnancy-related joint mobility has changed how these muscles fire, or weakness is making certain movements feel harder, we've just established that focused training around the pelvis may be essential for progressing through the Function phase of CFF. Let's make our way around the pelvis!

Adductors (Inner Thigh Muscles)

Your adductors, or inner thigh muscles, bring your legs toward the midline and help stabilize the pelvis during movements like squats, lunges, and single-leg exercises. They also share a direct connection with the pelvic floor muscles (PFM) since both attach to the pubic bone. Because of this, changes in pelvic floor strength or tension can influence adductor function. When the pelvic floor is weak, the adductors may become overactive, contributing to hip tightness, restricted mobility, or groin pain. Conversely, weak adductors can make movements like standing from a chair feel unstable or cause your knees to collapse inward during a squat.

Training Tips

Since the adductors and pelvic floor muscles are interconnected, I like a coordinated training approach. If your goal is to relax the pelvic floor, try doing so during inner thigh stretches. If you need to strengthen both the adductors and the pelvic floor, a great exercise is Pilates ball squeezes with pelvic floor contractions, either in a seated position or while performing a glute bridge, although current research does not yet show that co-training the hip muscles and PFM is more beneficial than training them separately.

Abductors (Glute Medius and Minimus)

Your abductors, the glute medius and minimus, are muscles on the outer hip and thigh that move your leg away from your body (think "abduct" as in "away") and play a key role in keeping your pelvis steady when you walk, lunge, or shift weight from one leg to another, preventing one side from dropping. During pregnancy, as your pelvis becomes more mobile and your center of gravity shifts forward, weak or underused abductors may struggle to provide stability, leading to hip discomfort or even a waddling gait. Carrying a baby on one side can put extra stress on one hip, causing the abductors on that side to work harder while the lower back compensates.

The piriformis, a deep hip stabilizer and external rotator, also helps control hip and pelvic movement. While it assists with hip abduction when your hip is flexed (like at the bottom of a squat), its main job is hip stability and external rotation. The piriformis can become tight or overactive, pressing on the sciatic nerve and causing symptoms similar to sciatica, including pain, numbness, or tingling in the glute and down the leg. This is known as piriformis syndrome, which is different from true sciatica, as it results from muscle compression rather than a spinal issue like a herniated disc.

Training Tip

You're probably familiar with exercises like lateral band walks and clam shells, which help strengthen the abductors, and flexibility exercises like figure four or pigeon that help stretch the hips. I also like to target the glute medius and minimus in functional roles like providing pelvic stability. One exercise I've used with moms (who don't have any SPD pain) is a single-leg Pilates ball press against the wall (leg lifted nearest the wall and with a ball at knee height, press the ball into the wall and hold). Additionally, I coach moms on how to enhance exercises like side-lying leg lifts by emphasizing pelvic stability by using a Pilates ball. I highly encourage you to try this as it's been a game changer for many moms, providing that "aha" moment when they finally feel the right muscles working. Here is what you do:

- Lie on your side with a Pilates ball placed between your waist and the floor, positioned just below your rib cage and above your hip bone.
- Keep your bottom leg bent for support while your top leg extends straight.
- As you lift your top leg with your toes pointed at the floor, focus on keeping your torso anchored to the ball. Avoid

shifting your pelvis to help lift the leg. Lower with control and repeat.

Pelvic Floor Muscles

We've already covered the role of the pelvic floor in core training, but since we're working our way around the pelvis they belong in this chapter as well. Early in the book, you learned how PFM coordinate with the diaphragm and transverse abdominis, and we also discussed how they can be incorporated into your strength training routine. In this chapter, we've touched on how they interact with the adductors, creating a co-relationship in function and dysfunction. Now, I'd like to provide a few tips if you are under the care of a pelvic floor physical therapist and targeting your PFM.

Training Tip

While coaching moms who are also seeing a pelvic floor physical therapist, here is what I've uncovered:

- Moms have a lot of responsibilities, and sometimes even a few simple exercises can feel like too much to incorporate into an already busy day. I've found that many moms choose between doing their "homework" PT exercises or working out. To stay consistent with both, I suggest you ask your physical therapist if you can integrate your isolation exercises into common strength exercises or stretches that are already a part of your fitness routine. Another approach would be to share the exercises you're already doing with your PT and ask if any of the assigned PT exercises are already being trained in your routine so that your PT can avoid prescribing redundant exercises.

- Similar to the first suggestion, if you do have assigned PT exercises and you're working with a personal trainer, share those exercises with the trainer or have your trainer connect with your physical therapist for collaboration. If your pelvic floor PT has you performing Kegels, your trainer could add a Pilates ball inner thigh squeeze with a Kegal to your hip thrusts or glute bridge. Or at the end of your session, your trainer could incorporate a happy baby pose to lengthen your PFM during your cooldown.

- Many people find it difficult to engage their glutes and to do so, many moms will just squeeze everything in an attempt to activate them, including PFM. If your PT exercises are meant to help you relax your pelvic floor muscles, then the last thing you want to do is excessively squeeze them during your workouts. Be mindful that you don't clench your PFM while training your glutes.

- Just like there are various training techniques to improve strength and tone in other muscles, you should change up your pelvic floor muscle training as well. If you're working on pelvic floor strength and endurance, you can vary the pace with strong, longer holds or gentle, quick flickers.

Hip Flexors (Psoas and Iliacus)

Your hip flexors, primarily the psoas and iliacus, are deep muscles at the front of your hips that connect your lower spine and pelvis to your thigh bone. They play a key role in lifting your legs, bending at the hips, and stabilizing your pelvis during movement. You rely on them constantly, whether you're walking, climbing stairs, or even just standing upright.

During pregnancy, as your belly grows, your center of gravity shifts forward, often increasing the curve in your lower back (lumbar lordosis) and tilting the pelvis forward (anterior pelvic tilt). This positioning can keep the psoas in a shortened position for long periods, contributing to discomfort or reduced mobility. At the same time, prolonged sitting, whether from feeding a baby, desk work, or driving, can have a similar effect, limiting hip extension and making it harder to move efficiently. In all cases, changes in hip flexor function can make movements like squats, lunges, and hip hinges feel more restricted or difficult to perform.

Training Tip

Since hip flexor mobility and strength are equally important, your training may need to address both. If your hip flexors feel tight, a half-kneeling hip flexor stretch can help improve hip extension, especially if you spend long hours sitting. If you need to strengthen them, banded standing marches are an effective way to improve control and function.

Upper Body

Strength (Lower Traps, Rhomboids, and Mid-Back)

Many moms develop a forward, rounded shoulder posture. To help prevent this, it's essential to strengthen the lower trapezius, rhomboids, and other mid-back muscles. The lower trapezius, located in the mid-to-lower back and attaching from the spine up to the bottom of the shoulder blade, helps pull the scapula downward and stabilize it during overhead movement. The rhomboids, which run between the spine and the inner edges of the shoulder blades, act more like retractors, pulling the shoulder blades back and together. When these muscles are underactive, the upper trapezius, which runs from the base of the skull to the top of the shoulders, often compensates. This compensation can create that familiar feeling of upper back or neck tightness. That discomfort is often blamed on "tight muscles," but just like hip discomfort isn't always caused by tight hip flexors, upper-body tension isn't always about flexibility either.

Training Tips

Exercises like scapular retractions, prone T/Y/I raises, and banded rows effectively target these muscles to improve posture and function. When performing these exercises, be mindful not to shrug your shoulders up toward your ears, a common sign that the upper traps are taking over. Instead, focus on drawing your shoulder blades together and gently down your back, as if you're tucking them into your back pockets. This helps activate the right muscles and reinforces the kind of movement that supports healthier posture and shoulder mechanics.

Mobility (Lats and Pecs)

Tight or overactive muscles can also interfere with movement patterns, especially when they restrict joint mobility or alter posture. For many moms, the latissimus dorsi and pectorals are common culprits.

The lats, which span from the lower back to the upper arm, influence shoulder extension and overhead mobility. The pectorals, located across the front of the chest, can shorten over time due to posture shifts and the repetitive forward positioning of daily tasks. When either of these muscles becomes restricted, it can limit thoracic extension, reduce shoulder range of motion, and disrupt the positioning needed for pushing and pulling movements.

Training Tips

Targeted mobility work, like lat foam rolling, chest openers, and thoracic extensions, can help release tension and restore range of motion. One of my favorite techniques is Pilates ball thoracic breathing, where you lie on your back with a small ball under your upper back near bra strap level and focus on expanding your rib cage with deep, diaphragmatic breaths. One benefit is that this counters forward-leaning postures. In addition, because the lats and chest muscles attach to the rib cage, restricted mobility in these areas can impact breathing mechanics. Diaphragmatic breathing can help release tension in both muscle groups. Lastly, when working on mobility, watch for excessive arching in the lower back, which often compensates for limited movement through the thoracic spine.

Do You Need Additional Support?

As mentioned in the introduction to this chapter, training movement patterns should be your functional strength training priority. However, if you're noticing difficulty in performing those compound exercises with good form, then strengthening and/or lengthening the muscles in this chapter could be just what you need. Additionally, if you're pregnant or postpartum, adding a few isolated exercises to your routine will help you adapt to the changes your body is going through. Lastly, if you're experiencing poor posture or discomfort at any stage of motherhood, please return to this chapter and begin troubleshooting (along with seeing a doctor if you're feeling pain).

Here are some sample exercises and brief descriptions to get you started:

Pelvic Floor Muscles

- Basic Kegel holds: Gently contract and lift the pelvic floor, hold for five to ten seconds, then fully release.
- Quick-flick Kegels: Quickly squeeze and release the pelvic floor muscles in rapid succession.
- Elevator Kegels: Engage the pelvic floor in stages, gradually increasing contraction as if an elevator is moving up, then lowering it back down.
- Diaphragmatic breathing: Inhale deeply, allowing the belly to expand and pelvic floor muscles to relax.
- Child's pose: Sit back onto heels with arms extended forward, focusing on fully relaxing the pelvic floor.
- Cat/cow: Inhale into the cow position with an arched back while fully releasing the pelvic floor; exhale into the cat position with a gentle engagement.

Adductors (Inner Thigh)

- Side-lying adductor lifts: Lie on your side and lift the straight bottom leg while keeping the foot flexed.
- Ball squeezes in bridge position: Squeeze a ball between the knees while performing a glute bridge.
- Seated butterfly stretches: Sit with the soles of your feet together, and gently let the knees fall toward the floor without bouncing.

- Copenhagen plank: Hold a side plank with the top leg supported on a bench, engaging your inner thighs for stability.
- Adductor slides on sliders: While in a partial squat, extend one leg outward on a sliding disc and control the return movement.
- Plie squat pulses: Stand with feet turned out and perform small, controlled pulses at the bottom of the squat.
- Cable machine adductions: Stand next to a cable machine and pull the leg inward against resistance, keeping the foot flexed.

Abductors and Piriformis

- Side-lying leg raises: Lie on your side and lift the top leg with the toe slightly pointed downward.
- Clamshells: Lie on your side with your knees bent, keep your feet together, and open your knees.
- Banded lateral walks: Step sideways while keeping tension in a resistance band around the feet, ankles, or above the knees.
- Standing hip abductions: Stand tall, hold onto support, and lift one leg outward without leaning.
- Fire hydrants: Start on hands and knees, lifting one knee out to the side at a 90-degree angle without rotating the hips.
- Side plank with leg lifts: Hold a side plank while lifting the top leg to challenge hip stability.
- Single-leg standing balance with Pilates ball press: Press a Pilates ball against a wall with your lifted knee while balancing on the opposite leg.
- Banded seated abductions: Sit upright with a resistance band above the knees and push the knees outward against resistance.

- Pigeon pose variations: Start in a lunge position, then lower the front shin toward the floor, aiming for a 45–90 degree angle, while keeping the back leg extended straight behind you and lowering the hips for a deep stretch.
- Figure-4 stretches: Lie on your back with both knees bent, cross one ankle over the opposite knee, then grab behind the bottom thigh and gently pull it toward your chest while keeping the top foot flexed.
- Seated piriformis stretches: Sit upright on a bench with both feet on the floor, cross one ankle over the opposite knee, then gently lean forward from the hips while keeping the top foot flexed to deepen the stretch.

Hip Flexors

- Half-kneeling hip flexor stretch: Start in a half-kneeling position with one knee on the floor and the other foot forward, tuck the tailbone under, and gently press the hips forward.
- Dynamic alternating lunge holds: Step into a deep lunge and hover the back knee just above the ground for a controlled hold.
- Banded march: Loop a resistance band around both feet, stand tall, and alternately lift each knee toward hip height while maintaining core stability.
- Hanging leg raises: Hang from a pull-up bar and lift your knees toward the chest while keeping the core engaged and movement controlled.

Lats/Lower Traps/Rhomboids

- Prone Y raises: Lie on your stomach with arms extended in a Y position, thumbs up and lift your arms off the floor.

- Prone T raises: Lie on your stomach with arms in a T position, palms facing feet, and lift your arms while keeping the chest down.

- Prone I raise: Lie on your stomach with arms extended overhead and lift your arms while keeping the neck neutral.

- Cable face pulls: Use a rope attachment to pull the cable toward your forehead while keeping elbows high and wide.

- Scapular retractions: Stand or sit with shoulders down and back, squeezing shoulder blades together.

- Band pull-apart: Hold a resistance band at chest level and pull it apart while keeping your arms straight.

- Lat foam rolling: Lie semi-sideways on a foam roller, rolling along the lat muscle while keeping the arm overhead.

- Wall "snow" angels: Stand against a wall and slowly raise and lower your arms like making a snow angel while keeping your back flat.

Chest (Pecs) Flexibility

- Doorway stretches: Place forearms on either side of a doorway and gently step forward to stretch the chest.

- Side-lying chest opener: Lie on your side with the top knee supported on a foam roller, and rotate the upper body open to stretch the chest.

- Seated clasp: Sit tall, interlace fingers behind the back, and pull the elbows wide while opening the chest.
- Pilates ball thoracic breathing: Lie with a Pilates ball at bra strap height, extend arms open to the sides, and take deep breaths to expand the chest.

Take Action

If you're ready to put this into practice, choose one of the following next steps:

1. Think about the major movement patterns that are the most challenging for you. Consider whether lack of mobility or weakness in these supporting muscles may be contributing to the challenge.
2. Review Appendix B for additional resources to support your targeted training.

9

When to Push, Pause, or Pivot

Key Insights from This Chapter

- There are trends during pregnancy and common predicaments postpartum that create uncertainty whether to pause, pivot, or push through exercise. With knowledge and strategy, most moms can stay physically active by progressing and regressing when necessary.
- Prenatal and postpartum exercise recommendations have typically been lumped together, but we now have more comprehensive guidance on the first year postpartum, so make sure you're relying on updated guidance.

Motherhood brings significant changes, not just to your body but also to how you think about exercise. If you're reading this, chances are you've experienced moments of uncertainty: wondering how hard to push, when to modify, or whether to pause altogether.

In my work with moms, I've seen these decision points come up repeatedly, moments where navigating fitness through motherhood feels confusing or even a little scary. These can be "make-or-break" moments. Times when you have to decide: Do I push forward? Do

I pause and wait? Or do I pivot and try something different? If you struggle to answer those questions, the default tends to be to pause or stop altogether, thinking you'll wait out the uncertainty and be more confident about exercise selection at another stage of motherhood.

This chapter goes beyond just the physical signs that tell you when to progress or scale back. We'll explore real-life situations and common questions that can feel overwhelming without clear guidance. Along the way, I'll offer insights to help you feel self-assured; even if I don't answer your exact question, you'll know to make informed choices that feel right for you.

You'll notice the guidance in this chapter is divided into three sections: Trimester Trends, Postpartum Predicaments, and Progression/Regression Strategies (helpful for all stages). Choose a section, and let's clear up those uncertainties!

Trimester Trends

You've probably noticed that most pregnancy books are organized by trimester. It's an easy way to find what feels most relevant at each stage, and it works well because most pregnancies tend to follow a similar timeline. However, it is my opinion that when it comes to pregnancy and exercise, although there are similarities in terms of what's happening to your body throughout pregnancy, there are too many unique fitness and lifestyle factors for me to feel comfortable providing specific advice based on trimester alone. The guidance in this chapter will be rooted in trimester "trends," but the differentiator is that rather than blanket advice, I will present factors that can help you know when to push forward or when to modify your training plan. In fact, if moms-to-be like Jade, Nadiya, or Haley had given in to the assumption that by the third trimester, they'd be too uncomfortable to do certain exercises or that they wouldn't be able to challenge their core after the first trimester, then they may not have gotten to their due date feeling stronger and more confident than ever before.

First Trimester Trends

During the first trimester, your body is undergoing hormonal changes that can have a rapid impact on your body, even very early on in pregnancy. Let's take a look at common questions associated with first trimester trends.

I'm Pregnant and Want to Exercise! Should I Speak to a Doctor First, or Not?

Before I answer this, let's consider where this question stems from, which is whether exercise can harm your baby. And because your baby's health is your number one priority, it's a valid question to ask. The overwhelming consensus is clear: physical activity during pregnancy decreases the risk of preeclampsia, hypertension, gestational diabetes, excessive weight gain, delivery complications, postpartum depression, and newborn complications. Additionally, physical activity has no adverse effects on birthweight or increased risk of stillbirth.[1] If your pregnancy is healthy and without complications, it's safe to continue, or even begin, an exercise routine. So, if these are the facts, why is exercise during pregnancy still such a common concern?

For starters, there's been a long-standing lack of research focused specifically on maternal exercise. Ethically, researchers haven't always studied the pregnancy and postpartum period (but we have some dedicated researchers and advocates in the field so that is changing). On top of that, professional organizations in fitness and obstetrics typically wait for a large body of evidence before releasing public guidelines. Even once those guidelines exist, outdated information continues to circulate, often long after the research has evolved. And with so much content living indefinitely online, it can take time for both moms and healthcare providers to become aware of what's actually current and evidence based. As a sidenote, that's why high-intensity exercise isn't being widely recommended or clearly outlined. It's not because we know it's unsafe but because there hasn't been enough research yet for guidelines to be updated. That said, small studies have shown that healthy pregnant women in their third trimester tolerated short bursts of high-effort exercise well. Even when heart rates were higher, there were no negative effects on fetal heart rate or blood flow, and all markers stayed within normal ranges.[2]

Earlier guidelines stated that previously inactive moms could begin exercising during pregnancy, under medical supervision. While not a direct prohibition, this cautious tone often led to the widespread belief that starting exercise during pregnancy wasn't safe unless you were already active. To further the fear and caution, exercise guidelines often lead with contraindications to exercise, or in other words, reasons not to exercise. Understanding these complications is important for your health and your baby's; however, it's important to note the distinction that exercise doesn't "cause" those conditions. In fact, leading maternal health researchers have put out a call to "re-evaluate clinical guidelines related to medical disorders that have previously been considered contraindications to prenatal exercise. Removing barriers to physical activity during pregnancy for women with certain medical conditions may in fact be beneficial for maternal–fetal health outcomes."[3]

To empower the majority of healthy moms-to-be to overcome any concerns they might have about getting or staying active, the Get Active Questionnaire for Pregnancy (GAQ-P) was developed. This assessment tool is designed to identify the small number of moms who need to consult with a healthcare professional before they begin or continue to be physically active. You can complete the four questions for your own reassurance, or if you're under the care of a doctor and feel more comfortable with guidance, you can complete the form with them.[4]

If you're discussing your plan to exercise with your doctor, be ready to advocate for yourself and ask for specific information if any cautious recommendations are provided to you. Some healthcare providers don't routinely offer physical activity guidance during pregnancy. Many may not even be familiar with current recommendations.[5] A helpful way to open the conversation with your doctor is to ask, "Do I have any contraindications or concerns that limit my ability to exercise?"

I realize I didn't exactly answer the question, but that's because if you're under the care of a health provider, nobody is going to tell you not to have that conversation. But, if you aren't able to obtain prenatal care, there are tools to guide you.

I'm Ready to Exercise! Do I Need to Start "Prenatal Exercise" or Not?

Yes, it's time to begin prenatal exercise. I don't want this to be all about semantics, but prenatal exercise simply means exercise during pregnancy. That said, I get why the term can feel misleading. It's often associated with gentle movements and modifications that might seem unnecessary early on, especially if you're still feeling strong and capable of performing your current fitness routine.

And I agree with that. Just because you're pregnant doesn't mean you have to immediately switch to low-intensity workouts or stop doing the exercises you were doing before. But here's how I look at it: prenatal exercise means following a program that helps your body adapt to the changes of pregnancy. And from that perspective, the earlier you start, the better. For example, adding targeted work for your pelvic floor or upper back isn't about scaling back, it's about building the strength and awareness that will support you as pregnancy progresses. That is "prenatal exercise." If you're wondering whether you should sign up for a prenatal class, the answer is: maybe. It depends on the class and the instructor. If the class still challenges you and doesn't require you to take on unnecessary modifications you don't need yet, it could be motivating and help with consistency, as well as an opportunity to connect with other moms-to-be.

Ugh, Now I Have Morning Sickness! Do I Try to Stick with My Fitness Plan, or Not?

For some of you, this will be a decision based on how bad you feel and what you can tolerate. For others with more severe cases of morning sickness, you might not have much say in the decision. If you're experiencing nausea, whether you continue to exercise could be a matter of scheduling adjustments. Take note of the time of day when you're least likely to experience "morning" sickness. Unless you're experiencing nausea all day, most moms notice a pattern. One solution is to temporarily adjust your workout schedule so that your activity takes place during the time of day when you're least likely to feel sick.

If morning sickness prevents you from eating or causes you to avoid specific foods, you may notice a dip in your energy levels. With less energy and fewer nutrients to support recovery, you may still be able to stay physically active, but you'll likely need to adjust the intensity and duration of your workouts. Exercise shouldn't make you feel more tired, and pushing through a workout at an intensity that doesn't match your energy certainly won't feel good or motivating.

Lastly, if your morning sickness is more severe and you're frequently vomiting, you'll also need to be mindful of dehydration. If you choose to stay active, make sure you're drinking enough fluids and avoiding hot or humid environments that could increase your risk of dehydration.

Second Trimester Trends

For many moms, the exhaustion felt during the first trimester begins to diminish, making establishing a steady workout schedule feel more attainable. However, changes to your body's major systems, like the cardiovascular, respiratory, and metabolic systems, continue. Let's review second trimester trends and how they may affect exercise, as well as how exercise can help you adapt to these changes.

My Heart Rate Is above 140 BPM. Should I Slow Things Down, or Not?

One of the most persistent myths in prenatal fitness is that your heart rate shouldn't go above 140 bpm (beats per minute) during pregnancy. Despite being removed from official guidelines in 1994, more than half of the healthcare providers surveyed still recommend this limit.[6] It's another example of how outdated information continues to circulate, even as our understanding of exercise during pregnancy has evolved. This book is about empowerment, so let me help you understand why hitting 140 bpm isn't an automatic indicator to dial it back or slow down.

Heart rate, the number of times your heart beats per minute, is a common way to measure exercise intensity or how hard your body is working. The more effort you put in, the more oxygen your muscles require and the faster your heart pumps. Exercise science has provided formulas to estimate your maximum heart rate and define zones for low, moderate, and vigorous intensity based on percentages of that maximum. This can be helpful when training for specific goals, and with wearables like watches and earbuds, tracking heart rate during a workout is more accessible than ever.

Now that you understand heart rate as a measure of intensity during exercise, it's important to know that heart rate monitoring may be less effective during pregnancy due to the changes in your cardiovascular system. Pregnancy demands more oxygen and nutrients, which means your body is going to produce more blood and your heart is going to beat faster to circulate it. An increased resting heart rate is a common indicator that this is happening. As a result of heart rate variability during pregnancy, heart rate monitors may underestimate intensity at higher effort levels and overestimate it at lower ones, making them less reliable tools.[7] An effective alternative measure of intensity is the talk test: if you can talk but you're unable to sing, you're likely working at a moderate intensity.

This supports why the 140 bpm limit is no longer included in current exercise guidelines for pregnancy. Additionally, while it was originally introduced as a cautious recommendation, it doesn't reflect what we now know about how advantageous exercise can be during uncomplicated pregnancies. In fact, recent studies have found vigorous-intensity exercise during healthy pregnancies, particularly in women who were active before pregnancy, to be safe. For example, women who continued high-intensity training throughout pregnancy improved their cardiovascular fitness (VO_2 max) from mid-pregnancy through the postpartum period, with no negative effects on their babies.[8] Vigorous exercise often corresponds to heart rates above 140 bpm, typically between 77 percent and 95 percent of your maximum heart rate, depending on your age and fitness level. A few small studies involving elite athletes have shown temporary changes in fetal heart rate or uterine blood flow immediately following very intense exercise, at 90 percent or more of max heart rate. However, these changes were resolved quickly and did not result in harm to the baby.

So, please don't be fearful if your heart rate goes above 140 bpm. Individualize your program so that you're working at an intensity level that is right for you, and monitor that intensity based on how hard you feel you're working (talk test).

I Feel So Out of Shape! Do I Need to Exercise More, or Not?

During the second trimester, you may notice changes in your breathing due to both hormonal shifts and the physical growth of your baby. As the uterus expands, it begins to push the diaphragm and nearby organs upward, giving the lungs less room to fully empty, with up to 70 percent of pregnant moms reporting feeling more short of breath during everyday activities. The good news is that your body adapts in smart ways. The rib cage widens and shifts in shape to help preserve total lung capacity (keeping your breathing rate generally unchanged), and you start taking deeper breaths. You actually become more efficient at taking in and using oxygen to meet the increasing needs of both you and your baby.[9]

Another factor that may contribute to you feeling "out of shape" may be due to the changes in your upper airways. Increased levels of estrogen and progesterone can cause more blood flow and swelling in the nasal tissues, often leading to a feeling of congestion or stuffiness. These changes, combined with deeper breathing, can make the sensation of shortness of breath more pronounced for some moms.[10]

So, if you're maintaining an exercise program, don't assume these respiratory changes mean you're out of shape or need to push harder to improve fitness. That said, if you're not exercising consistently, it could be contributing to how you're feeling, and adding more movement to your routine may help.

My Bump Is Getting Bigger. Should I Start Eating for Two, or Not?

This question isn't directly about exercise, but it does relate to changes in metabolism and common concerns around weight gain that are more prevalent in the second trimester, so it's a helpful place to start the conversation.

Your metabolism shifts during pregnancy to support your growing baby. Your metabolic system is responsible for converting the food you eat into energy your body can use. During pregnancy, this system works harder, and the amount of energy (calories) your body uses even while resting (basal metabolic rate) increases to support the growth and development of your baby. This metabolic change is one of the reasons you might feel hungrier or more tired than usual. Although you may need to consume more calories to use for energy, this doesn't equate to what you may think of when you hear "eating for two." In fact, much of the weight you gain during pregnancy, like increased blood volume, muscle, placenta, and amniotic fluid, requires surprisingly little additional energy. As a result, your daily calorie needs increase only modestly during the second and third trimesters, an additional 340 calories during the second trimester and about 450 additional daily calories during the third trimester.[11]

From an exercise perspective, if you've been told to increase your calorie intake to meet daily energy needs, it's important to also factor in the additional energy required for physical activity. This might require a bit of a mindset shift, especially if, before pregnancy, you viewed exercise primarily as a way to "burn" calories. A practical way to support your workouts is by eating a small protein and carbohydrate snack thirty to ninety minutes beforehand. This can help maintain your energy during exercise and help you recover afterward. Here are a few options:

- Greek yogurt or cottage cheese with berries
- Whole grain toast with peanut butter and banana
- Cheese and whole grain crackers
- Oatmeal with toppings like nuts or fruit

So, should you start eating for two? Not quite. While your body is doing more, your energy needs go up gradually, not drastically. Additionally, your energy needs may be different from someone else's depending on several factors, including your starting weight and body composition, so you should work with your doctor or a registered dietitian to tailor those recommendations to your unique body and pregnancy.

My Arms Look Flabby. Should I Exercise to Burn More Calories, or Not?

Pregnant or not, every body type is different, and when fat is gained, you can't control where it's stored or choose which areas your body pulls from for energy. That means you can't target fat loss in your arms or any other specific spot.[12] But more importantly, as you learned earlier, fat storage during pregnancy is purposeful; it helps build the reserves needed to support your baby's growth and prepare for breastfeeding.

So, while the short answer to this question is no, you shouldn't exercise more to "burn" calories or fat, I want to take it a step further and explain how exercise does play a role in how your body metabolizes calories and stores fat during pregnancy. Understanding this connection can help reframe how you view physical activity, not as a way to control appearance but as a way to support your body's function through all the changes happening.

During the second and third trimesters, hormonal shifts, including increases in human placental lactogen, cortisol, estrogen, and progesterone, make your body more resistant to insulin. Insulin is the hormone that helps move glucose (sugar) from your bloodstream into your cells to be used as energy. In pregnancy, this resistance is in some ways an intentional adaptation as it allows more glucose to remain in the bloodstream, so it can be delivered to your baby. Insulin also influences how your body stores fat. Increased insulin resistance can make your body more likely to store fat beyond what it actually needs.

So how does this tie into exercise? For starters, glucose (food broken down into sugar) is your body's preferred energy source for most types of physical activity. If your ability to use glucose efficiently is reduced, your body starts relying more on fat as fuel. That shift is another smart adaptation, but your body isn't automatically great at using fat efficiently.

That's where movement matters. If you perform moderate-intensity exercise, you can improve your ability to use fat as fuel, both during and after activity.[13] This means you'll have more energy for your workouts, support healthy weight gain, and be less likely to store excess fat in your arms or anywhere else. This is a big reason why I see exercise as a tool not to "burn calories" but to improve metabolic flexibility and the ability to use glucose and fat efficiently. Expecting moms who exercise have better-regulated insulin, which positively impacts weight management.

I'm Worried about My Glucose Test. Will Exercise Prevent Gestational Diabetes, or Not?

It might. Now that you understand the reasons behind insulin resistance during pregnancy, it's also important to know that this shift in increased blood sugar or glucose levels increases your body's need for insulin to keep blood sugar levels within a healthy range. To assess your body's ability to do this, your doctor will typically have you take a glucose screening between twenty-four and twenty-eight weeks of pregnancy. If your risk for gestational diabetes is higher due to risk factors like prior gestational diabetes, family history of diabetes, high blood pressure, PCOS, being overweight, or if you're over the age of thirty-five, the test may be ordered sooner.

The screening involves drinking a sweetened liquid, which contains 50 grams of sugar. A blood sample is taken one hour after drinking the solution to measure how the glucose was processed by your body. A higher-than-normal blood glucose level after sixty minutes means your provider will order a second glucose test to diagnose gestational diabetes. Every year, 2–10 percent of expecting moms in the United States are affected by gestational diabetes.[14]

Regular physical activity is one of the most effective ways to lower your risk of developing gestational diabetes, especially if you begin before pregnancy or even before conception. For moms diagnosed with gestational diabetes, exercise is not only safe, but it can also positively impact both blood sugar levels and overall pregnancy outcomes. Evidence shows that aerobic exercise lowers fasting and post-meal blood sugar, along with A1c levels. If you strength train, it can further improve your glucose control and may reduce the amount of insulin required if you use insulin therapy.[15]

Third Trimester Trends

The third trimester brings a continuation of many of the cardiovascular, metabolic, hormonal, and respiratory changes from the first and second trimesters, and many third trimester trends can be linked to the size and position of your baby. Let's explore some of them.

I'm Scared I Have Diastasis Recti. Should I Keep Training My Core, or Not?

Yes, keep training for core strength and function! As we covered earlier, abdominal separation is common in the third trimester as your belly expands. I remember a time when Louise arrived at the Active Mom Fitness studio for a session and anxiously asked if we should still be doing core exercises. The night before, she had noticed coning (a visible bulge or ridge along the midline of her stomach) as she was getting out of the bath. I reminded her that the linea alba, the connective tissue down the center of the abdomen, naturally stretches and thins as pregnancy progresses. In the third trimester, it's not unusual to see that thinning become visible, especially during movements that challenge core stability or create outward pressure. What you're seeing is the pressure from everything your belly is supporting pressing through that stretched centerline.

If this happens to you, don't panic, but don't ignore it either. Think of it as your body's way of saying: Let's adjust how we're moving. Use strategies like exhaling on exertion or rolling to your side before sitting up in bed to better manage pressure during everyday movements. And if you're feeling unsure or want more personalized support, a pelvic floor therapist can help you with additional strategies tailored to your body.

Next, we revisited a few of the core exercises Louise had been doing during her second trimester. With the growth of her belly in the third trimester, those same movements now triggered more obvious signs of abdominal separation. I reassured her, again, that some stretching of the linea alba at this stage is normal. But that didn't mean we needed to keep doing exercises that repeatedly stressed her abdomen in a way that produced visible symptoms. So, we made a few simple swaps and restructured her circuit.

We kept the focus on stability during push movements but traded TRX chest presses for stability ball wall push-ups (less pressure because of less gravitational pull). And instead of switching between standing, seated, and floor-based exercises throughout the circuit, I grouped exercises by position to minimize transitions that increase strain on the abdominal wall. Louise continued strength training until her due date and had no issues with diastasis recti after her postpartum healing.

Sometimes Physical Activity Is Painful. Should I Keep Exercising, or Not?

For you athletes or supermoms out there, you should not push through pain during your workouts. With your joints becoming more lax, your risk of discomfort increases. Core training will continue to support these changes, but some of you, despite your best efforts, will still experience SI joint pubic pain. For some moms, minor adjustments to the exercises you're performing are enough to reduce discomfort, but for others, it can be quite debilitating, and you may have to change your workout plans considerably. Small adjustments could mean avoiding single-leg exercises, where larger changes might mean non-weight-bearing cardio like recumbent bikes instead of long walks. If you're dealing with severe or disruptive pain, I hope you're working with a pelvic floor physical therapist who specializes in this area, so they can help you make exercise choices that support your recovery. Pain is not something you need to push through.

My Due Date Is Approaching! Should I Stop Exercising, or Not?

In short, no, there's no evidence to support stopping at a specific week of pregnancy. In fact, some of the most memorable and meaningful moments in my coaching experience happen during those final weeks. I have to say, one of my favorite parts about training moms-to-be is when we get close to the end of their pregnancy and start counting down the days to their due date. It's obviously an exciting time, they're about to meet their baby, but it's also a meaningful moment to acknowledge what their commitment to exercise has meant to them. It's always an honor for me to be part of that journey, and I feel lucky to have watched so many moms celebrate their strength in these final weeks.

Over the years, I've also gotten pretty good at noticing when a mom doesn't have many workouts left before labor begins. I've even predicted a few times when it was going to be the last workout because labor was near, mostly because I've noticed a kind of slowing down that goes beyond just feeling tired or having an "off" day. It's more like moving through a workout in slow motion. That may not be an evidence-based observation, but it's definitely a trend I've witnessed.

Because of that, I typically plan sessions with lower-intensity exercise and increased mobility work around thirty-seven weeks. In general, my goal at this point in the third trimester is to help moms maintain the strength they've already built and to stay physically active and mobile. Keep in mind that there is no exact number of weeks where this should occur, and that is why we also pay attention to other cues the body provides, like exercise recovery. If a mom starts feeling more tired or sore after workouts, that's a sign to adjust intensity or volume. Labor is a physical event, and the last thing I want is for someone to head into it feeling depleted from a workout.

For many moms, getting closer to their due date can also bring emotional and mental shifts, whether that's stress, anxiousness, or anticipation. So, I often shift the structure of workouts to include more stretching and opportunity for mindfulness. Extending the cooldown, adding pelvic floor relaxation exercises, or simply creating time to slow down can go a long way in helping a mom stay in the moment and increase feelings of calm and readiness.

So, to reiterate, approaching your due date doesn't mean you should stop exercising but to remind yourself that exercise is a powerful tool during pregnancy. If you need to make changes to pace, intensity, and exercise selection as you get closer to meeting your little one, then please do so.

Postpartum Predicaments

At the very beginning of this book, I shared my perspective on what postpartum means. It's often defined as the period immediately following childbirth, and terms like the fourth trimester are commonly used. As we move into this next section, I want to remind you not to feel bound by a specific timeline. I may refer to weeks, because much of the research does, but those weeks don't necessarily start the day you gave birth for all moms. Timelines will vary based on healing and recovery, so this isn't meant to be a rigid guide.

On a personal note, I'm especially excited to include this section because postpartum is finally being recognized as a distinct and important phase, not just an extension of pregnancy. For too long, prenatal and postpartum care have been lumped together, with recovery after birth treated as an afterthought. But that's starting to change. For the first time, guidelines have been developed specifically for the postpartum year, offering evidence-based recommendations on physical activity, sedentary behavior, and sleep.[16] These guidelines were created by a panel of researchers, healthcare providers, and exercise professionals, using both high-quality research and input from postpartum individuals (I had the opportunity to contribute to that early input phase!). It's an encouraging and long overdue shift toward giving postpartum care the focused attention it deserves. Let's explore some real-life questions and situations that may make you pause, give you confidence to push forward, or signal it's time to pivot.

I Just Had a Baby, You Want Me to Move Already?

I'll never forget the pain I felt as the nurses encouraged me to walk the hospital halls or how swollen my feet were, so much so that I couldn't even fit into the shoes I came in wearing. In the early days to weeks postpartum, your body is managing a full spectrum of recovery: uterine cramping, lochia (postpartum bleeding), hormonal shifts, perineal or incision soreness, breast engorgement, and swelling. Many moms also experience fatigue, digestive changes, and a roller coaster of emotions. With all of that happening at once, it makes sense that movement doesn't feel like a top priority.

But here's the nuance: movement and exercise aren't the same thing. Light activity, like short walks, breathing exercises, or pelvic tilts, can actually support recovery, improve circulation, and reduce the risk of blood clots, even within the first few days postpartum. The key is that it's supportive and restorative. Healing takes precedence, but physical activity can serve as one element that facilitates this process.

In the first two weeks, this might look like walking around your house, diaphragmatic breathing, and using proper body mechanics when lifting your baby. If around two to four weeks, you're feeling ready, you can begin light core reengagement, like pelvic floor contract-and-relax work or breathing with gentle abdominal activation. You may even be able to tolerate longer walks of five to ten minutes. If this activity doesn't produce symptoms, around weeks five and six, you could try low-load functional movements like sit-to-stands.[17]

I've Been Cleared, Now What?

That six-week checkup often feels like a big milestone, but that's because that traditionally has been the only postpartum care visit you get. It's when your provider either gives you the green or red light to resume physical activity and sex.

Let's first discuss what being cleared actually means. During your postpartum visit, your doctor will check in to see how you are adapting to life with your baby and evaluate how your body is healing after labor and delivery. Clearance usually indicates that your uterus is shrinking, any tearing or incisions have healed, and no immediate medical concerns are preventing you from becoming more active. What it doesn't always assess is your pelvic floor function, core coordination, nutritional intake, or mental readiness for exercise. Yet all of those directly affect your ability to continue healing and tolerate increased activity. In other words, clearance is just one piece of the puzzle and directly tied to the scope of your provider's medical expertise, not necessarily a full picture of your physical readiness.

Healing doesn't end at six weeks.[18] While external healing may be visible, deep recovery is still underway. Research shows that pelvic floor muscles stretched during delivery may take up to four to six months to fully recover their strength and function. Even after a cesarean birth, the uterine scar continues remodeling well past the six-week mark. In other words, it's not just okay to take your time, it's appropriate. If you're feeling ready to begin moving more intentionally, you can start with the CFF approach, which is designed to meet you where you are and help you build a strong foundation that supports your body as it continues to heal.

My message is to not do too much, too fast, too soon. That may not resonate with all of you. Some moms will hesitate to exercise because they're unsure of what to do or scared that they'll do something wrong. As I've said before, there's a fear culture around maternal exercise, so it isn't your fault that you feel this way. And hopefully, that will keep shifting as more research continues to challenge outdated limits. If you are cleared, your provider is letting you know there is no absolute contraindication for exercise, meaning nothing specific is going to cause you harm because of a medical condition. If you don't have any medical concerns holding you back, returning to physical activity within the first twelve weeks after birth is not only safe but also ideal.[19] Movement supports both your physical recovery and your mental well-being, and both are essential. For a quick mental check-in, you can also consider things like:

- Does exercise feel like a stressor, or are you feeling excited to get back into a routine?
- Does your energy feel depleted after increased movement?
- Do you feel emotionally ready and supported, or does the idea of exercise feel overwhelming?

I Don't Want to Decrease My Milk Supply

If you're wondering if exercise will interfere with your milk supply, fortunately, it does not. If you're enjoying moderate-intensity exercise, your body is capable of producing the same amount of milk, with the same nutrients, as nonexercising moms. Babies of moms who exercise gain weight appropriately and haven't experienced adverse effects on feeding.[20] During high-intensity workouts, the taste of your breastmilk might alter slightly, but it's not harmful to your baby and seems to only last about an hour.

Now, just because science says exercise doesn't impact breastfeeding, that doesn't mean there aren't practical challenges during the early months, especially when your schedule revolves around your baby's feeding schedule. It may take a little more strategy, like breastfeeding right before a workout so that exercise is more comfortable, and you buy yourself some time or choose home workouts to lessen the time away from your baby (that way you're not spending your precious fitness time away worrying if the baby is hungry). One more practical consideration is in your sports bra. With your breasts being larger, it's probably best to opt for the most supportive bra, which would be high-impact bras, usually with wide straps or racerback style. Nursing bras are not going to be supportive enough for anything beyond light movement. I personally liked the sports bras that had a front closure so that if I did need to feed my daughter before having a chance to change, it was easier access.

Finally, keep in mind that breastfeeding increases your calorie and hydration needs, so make sure you're fueling enough to support both recovery and milk production. Because it's great to consume carbohydrates and protein after a moderate to vigorous workout, consider making a post-workout snack part of your post-workout breastfeeding routine. In conclusion, it may not always be easy, but breastfeeding doesn't mean pausing physical activity.

I've Heard Exercise Can Help with Postpartum Depression

It can. Postpartum depression (PPD) affects many new mothers and can develop anytime in the first year after birth. It's more than mood swings; symptoms may include persistent sadness, low energy, anxiety, trouble bonding with your baby, or feelings of hopelessness. If you're reading this before you've had your baby, one thing I suggest is having a transparent and informative conversation with the people in your inner circle, whether a spouse, friend, or family member. I encourage you to discuss the possibility of postpartum depression and ask them to keep an eye out for symptoms they may notice within you that you may not see. You could take it a step further and seek out PPD support resources during pregnancy so that if it does occur, you and your trusted circle aren't having to do that while also caring for a baby.

In addition to clinical mental health support, exercise helps prevent and reduce symptoms of postpartum depression. Exercise increases mood-related neurotransmitters like serotonin and dopamine, and helps regulate sleep, energy, and cognitive function. It also reduces inflammatory markers, which are frequently elevated in postpartum depression.[21] The most effective programs tend to involve moderate-intensity activity, done three to five times per week, but even lower-intensity movement can help you.[22]

Don't get hung up on specifics. Walking, strength training, aerobic workouts, and yoga have all been used successfully. The important thing is to start moving. If you're reading this while still pregnant, there's also evidence that regular exercise during pregnancy can lower your risk of developing postpartum depression. So, wherever you are on the journey, consider exercise a proven tool for your mental wellness (see Appendix B for mental health resources).

To Nap or Workout, That Is the Question

This heading is a bit simplified. The real question is whether, while sleep-deprived, you should prioritize exercise or wait until you're getting more rest to push through a workout. Because exercise is a stressor to your body (albeit a positive one) and sleep deprivation also stresses your body, it's important to consider how the stress of both might affect you.

On the one hand, exercise can improve energy levels and sleep quality, which probably sounds wonderful to you if you're not getting much sleep. On the other hand, lack of sleep can compromise exercise recovery, increase how hard your workout feels, lead to poor pelvic floor recovery, and interfere with the results you're working toward. Let's take a closer look at how sleep and exercise interact, so you can make a more informed decision on pausing, pivoting, or pushing through a workout.

During strength workouts, your muscles experience microtears, and it's during recovery, especially sleep, that they then repair so that your muscles are stronger or more defined. Growth hormone, one of the key hormones involved in this repair process, is primarily released during deep sleep. If you're regularly missing out on quality sleep, your muscles may not have the time or resources to recover, even if your workouts are consistent. So, if you choose to work out, make sure you're also setting yourself up for a good night's sleep to support recovery, or adjust your workout goals so that intensity, recovery, and results are better aligned with the rest you're getting at this stage of motherhood.

Sleep deprivation also affects how hard exercise feels, or your "perceived exertion." If your usual routine suddenly feels more difficult, it might not be your fitness level, it might be your lack of sleep causing your training session to feel more difficult. That can lead to frustration and lack of confidence and motivation. Interestingly, studies suggest that short-interval workouts, especially intervals under thirty seconds, may feel more manageable during sleep-deprived states compared to longer bouts of effort. So, if you're committed to being consistent in your fitness routine, try adjusting the structure of your workout to change your perceived exertion.

If you're postpartum and ready to tackle weight, don't forget how important sleep is in the process, too. Your body uses hormones to help control hunger, fullness, stress, and even fat storage. Two of these hormones, leptin and ghrelin, help tell your brain when you're full or hungry. But when you're sleep-deprived, those signals get mixed up, making you feel extra hungry and craving more high-carb or sugary foods.

Another key hormone is cortisol, your body's stress hormone. When you don't get enough sleep, cortisol can stay high, which tells your body to hold onto fat, especially around your belly. It can also make it harder to sleep the next night.

This doesn't mean you shouldn't exercise for weight loss, but again, if you're not getting enough sleep, it can be really discouraging to keep pushing through workouts for weight loss despite feeling fatigued and not seeing results. Choosing to be physically active instead of taking a nap might be what your body needs, but in my opinion, I wouldn't suggest weight loss being your motivation for activity if your sleep isn't supporting it yet.

So, what about napping instead? Short naps, even just twenty to forty minutes, can boost your focus, memory, and how well your body performs, especially if you didn't sleep well the night before.[23] The best time to nap is between 1:00 and 4:00 in the afternoon. If you're just dealing with a rough night here or there, it might help to move your workout earlier in the day. And if you can fit in both a workout and a nap, try to keep that afternoon nap window open.

Although the nap or exercise predicament is common, the message here is really about sleep and physical activity. Continuing to balance sleep and physical activity for improved health outcomes is worth it, as they both have mental and physical benefits. Interestingly, when moms were given support or strategies to improve sleep, whether for themselves *or* their babies, they had fewer symptoms of depression.[24] Getting enough rest might feel out of reach, but it's not just a luxury; it's a powerful tool for healing.

To wrap up this section on postpartum predicaments, here are a few additional signs to help you determine if you should push, pause, or pivot.

Physical Signs to Consider Taking Pausing or Pivoting

- Muscle soreness lasting more than two days or taking longer to recover between workouts
- Feeling more fatigued than energized after exercise

Mental/Emotional Signs to Consider Pausing or Pivoting

- Mood changes or unusual irritability
- Exercise feels like stress rather than stress reliever
- Extreme fatigue throughout the day

Physical Signs to Consider Pushing Forward

- You're making progress and feeling good
- You're consistently fueling your body with enough calories and protein to support your activity level

Mental/Emotional Signs to Consider Pushing Forward

- You're feeling motivated and excited to take on more
- Your sleep is relatively consistent and restorative, even if not perfect

Progression and Regression Strategies

This last section is about adjusting exercise variables like pace, resistance, and position to meet your body where it's at, or in more training terms, "progress or regress." These strategies are helpful for moms at all stages of motherhood. My goal isn't to overwhelm you with technical details, but I do want you to see that unless you've hit a make-or-break moment where stopping is the best choice, there are plenty of ways to pivot, so you can stay consistent while still meeting your body's needs in the moment. You can adjust these training elements for a single session on days when you're low on energy or to advance your fitness plan when it's time to challenge yourself more.

Here are the essential exercise variables that help personalize any workout program. I've used the squat exercise to further explain what manipulating each variable looks like in practice.

Range of Motion

Range of motion or ROM refers to how much movement a joint can achieve in a specific direction during an exercise. For instance, when squatting, you may consider your thighs parallel to the floor a standard squat (90-degree bend in your knees). However, by going lower than that into a deeper squat, you're closer to the full range of motion and demand more of your ankles, knees, and hip joints as well as the muscles supporting them. I'm not advocating for one position over the other, but I'm sharing this so you can understand that changing the depth of the squat, or ROM, is one way to progress or regress this exercise based on your ability and needs. My client Helen was experiencing swelling in her ankles, not due to her pregnancy, but due to hardware that needed to come out after a surgery. To prevent further aggravation, we limited the range of motion in her squats so that she could continue to do them, even if not at the depth she was used to (at least until her surgery).

Base of Support

Your base of support is the area under your body that includes every point in contact with the ground, like the space between your two feet in a squat. If you're squatting with your feet wider than hip distance apart, your base of support is wider than if your feet were directly under your hips. A wider base, like in plié squat or sumo squats, provides you with greater stability and makes balancing easier in comparison to a narrow squat or a single-leg pistol squat. By changing your stance or base, you can make an exercise more or less challenging. For example, as you return to exercise postpartum, you may find it more appropriate to do wider-stance squats until your core strength and balance improve.

Aside from the impact your base of support has on exercise difficulty, it is a variable that can help manage discomfort as well. I worked with someone who has pudendal neuralgia, a pelvic nerve condition. Squats were an exercise she avoided because they typically caused pain. However, I knew she needed to master this movement pattern since it's so prevalent in daily life. Together, we learned that by pointing her toes inward slightly while narrowing the stance just an inch didn't increase pain! Can you imagine what this must have meant for someone who avoided exercise because it exacerbated her symptoms? So, although the squat didn't cure the pain, it didn't make it worse, and she was able to build the strength to incorporate other activities into her life again, like dance.

Tempo

Tempo is the speed and rhythm of each exercise movement, including how slowly you lower the weight, whether you pause, and how quickly you lift it back up. For example, adding a pause at the bottom of a squat increases the challenge compared to immediately standing back up. Tempo is interesting because both increasing and decreasing the speed of a squat can feel like you've added more challenge. It's a helpful way to adapt your home workout if you don't have access to heavier dumbbells or if you're short on time and can't get your normal three sets in, so you opt to feel the burn at a quicker pace.

Rest Intervals

Rest intervals are simply the recovery time you take between sets of exercises. For example, if you're performing bodyweight squats of fifteen repetitions, you might take a thirty- to sixty-second break between sets for your muscles to recover. This allows you time to rebuild the energy needed for a strong second set. Typically, shorter breaks are used for bodyweight or light weight endurance sets, while longer rest periods (two to three minutes) are better suited for heavy resistance or plyometric (jump) squats. If during your first trimester you were doing heavy smith machine squats, resting two minutes between sets, and then decide to decrease the weight you're squatting during your second trimester, you'd want to decrease the rest interval as well to maintain the same level of challenge.

As a sidenote, if you are lifting heavier weights, please don't overlook the rest period. Your body uses different energy systems to fuel your workouts, and when you're aiming for strength gains, that energy system needs time to replenish and fuel your next set. If you're someone who loves fitness classes, you're probably used to continuous movement with little rest, so it may feel like cheating to take a full three-minute recovery. I can't tell you how many groups I taught where this was the case. There were always a few moms picking their weights back up before our rest interval was over. However, I also know that busy moms are squeezing in quick workouts, so if you can't spare longer rest periods, try supersets like alternating between chest presses and squats so that your legs recover while your upper body is working.

Volume

I don't love math equations, but this one's simple, so don't skip it just because you see numbers. Training volume is the total amount of work you're doing in a workout. At its most basic, that could mean how many reps you perform in total. For example, if you do 3 sets of 10 squats, that's 30 total reps. But if you're using weight (like dumbbells), volume is often calculated as: weight × reps × sets. So, if you're holding 20 lbs. while doing those 3 sets of 10 squats: 20 × 10 × 3 = 600. Your total volume would be 600 pounds lifted for that exercise.

Understanding volume gives you a powerful tool; you can dial your workouts up or down by adjusting how much total work your body is doing, without having to rewrite your entire routine. If you're in your third trimester and feeling more fatigued and maybe not recovering as quickly from your workouts, you don't have to stop squatting altogether. You can reduce your volume by decreasing the weight, the number of reps, or even doing fewer sets. Instead of 3 sets of 10 with 20 lbs. (600 volume), you might do 2 sets of 8 with 15 lbs.: 15 × 8 × 2 = 240. You're doing the same movement, just less overall demand, which might get you back to the recovery timeline you're aiming for.

Load

Load refers to any kind of resistance your body has to work against. That can be your own bodyweight, added weight like dumbbells or barbells, or even resistance from tools like bands or suspension trainers (like a TRX). A bodyweight squat uses your body as the load. A goblet squat adds load by holding a dumbbell at your chest. A barbell back squat adds even more load by placing weight across your upper back. By adapting the load, you can scale your workout up or down when needed.

Now that you understand how to adjust key variables, the following chart provides examples of how this might look in practice for each of the major movement patterns. Refer to it in the way that works best for you. You could use it to:

- Create your own workouts: Build a circuit by selecting one exercise from each category. Keep in mind that you may not be on the same progression step for every category.

- Adapt a fitness app workout: Use the chart to substitute exercises that feel too advanced or not challenging enough. For instance, if the app suggests a stationary lunge but you want a greater challenge, you can progress to a forward or walking lunge.

- Modify movements in group classes: If your core isn't quite strong enough to sustain three sets of bent-over dumbbell rows, try for one set and then dial it back to a single-arm supported dumbbell row. You're still working the same major muscle groups and not risking injury.

Progression examples for major movement patterns (push, pull, squat, lunge)

	Progression 1	Progression 2	Progression 3	Progression 4	Progression 5
Push	Wall push-up (basic bodyweight, upright position)	Incline push-up (hands elevated on bench)	Knee push-up on floor (lowered base, more resistance)	Full push-up (floor, core engaged)	Push-up with tempo or band resistance (increased load/time under tension)
Pull	Seated resistance band row (basic position, controlled pull)	TRX or band-assisted standing row (slightly reduced support)	Single-arm dumbbell row (supported on bench)	Bent-over dumbbell row (more gravity)	Renegade row (plank position, anti-rotation demand)
Squat	Sit to stand (wide base, low depth)	Bodyweight squat (reduced height, narrow stance)	Goblet squat (added load, controlled descent)	Barbell back squat (greater load, upright posture)	Jump squat (power, fast tempo)
Lunge	Supported split squat (hands on wall, wide stance)	Static lunge (bodyweight, hands-free)	Reverse lunge (dynamic, core stability challenge)	Walking lunge (reduced base, forward movement)	Seesaw lunge (dynamic balance)

Progression examples for major movement patterns (vertical hinge, horizontal hinge, anti-rotation/rotation)

	Progression 1	Progression 2	Progression 3	Progression 4	Progression 5
Vertical Hinge	Hip hinge with dowel (body awareness + neutral spine)	Kettlebell deadlift (load with form control)	Romanian deadlift (hamstring-focused, hip control)	Single-leg RDL (balance + load control)	Single-leg RDL with tempo (eccentric load control)
Horizontal Hinge	Glute bridge (supine, minimal load)	Glute bridge with band or feet elevated (increased challenge)	Hip thrust (loaded, against bench)	Single-leg hip thrust (unilateral control and power)	Elevated hip thrust with band and weight (advanced glute challenge)
Anti-Rotation/Rotation	Supine knee drops/ seated trunk rotation (basic core engagement/ upright position)	Bird dog/ tall kneeling band press-out (stability + anti-rotation)	Dead bug with heel taps/ standing band press-out (core + control)	Half-kneeling band chop/ standing band rotation (transverse core work)	Standing cable chop with tempo/ rotational med ball throw (core + power)

Every season of motherhood brings new challenges, and with them, new decisions about how to move. The more you understand how to push, pause, or pivot with intention, the more confident you'll feel adjusting your workouts to meet your body's needs. Keep using these tools to stay consistent with your exercise goals, even when everything else is constantly changing.

Take Action

Whether you read the entire chapter or just the sections that applied most to your stage of motherhood, you should be able to finish this section with a clear action step in mind. Choose one of the following:

- If relevant, see Appendix B for resources on postpartum guidelines and training progressions during the first twelve months postpartum.
- Refer to the progression/regression chart the next time you're feeling stuck in a workout or you're facing the trends of pregnancy and predicaments postpartum.

Part IV

10

What about Cardio?

> **Key Insights from This Chapter**
>
> 1. Cardio is part of the Fitness component in the Core, Function and Fitness model. Its physical and mental health benefits are significant, but many forms of cardio are most effective, and better tolerated, once your core is functional and your muscles are strong.
>
> 2. Clear guidance exists for returning to running, emphasizing that tissue healing takes time after birth, hip and core strength are essential, and several other factors should be considered before reintroducing it into your routine.

In this chapter, we will shift our discussion to aerobic (cardiovascular) exercise and touch a bit more on mobility and flexibility. Both are components of the health and exercise guidelines and are recommended as part of a balanced fitness program.

In the Core, Function and Fitness method, mobility and flexibility are integral to the function component, as discussed in earlier chapters. Cardio resides at the top of the fitness pyramid, not due to a lack of value but because during and after pregnancy, reestablishing core strength and functional movement takes precedence. Once these foundational elements are solid, moms tend to find that incorporating other fitness aspects like cardio becomes more feasible.

Cardio or Aerobic?

Let's start with clarifying terminology and definitions. Cardio (short for cardiovascular) and aerobic are often used to mean the same thing, and for the most part, they are. Both involve steady movement that raises your heart rate and breathing, like walking, cycling, or dancing. While "aerobic" refers to how your body produces energy with oxygen, and "cardio" highlights the benefits to your heart, they overlap so much that most people (even experts) use the terms interchangeably. As a sidenote, resistance training is considered primarily *an*aerobic because it uses energy systems that don't depend on oxygen the same way.

Group fitness classes also fall under the aerobic category because they keep you moving continuously at a moderate to high intensity. Classes like spin, kickboxing, Zumba, and many forms of HIIT are designed to elevate your heart rate and keep it there, improving endurance and heart health over time.

What Really Happens to Your Physical Health When You're Consistent with Cardio?

Aerobic exercise sets off a chain of powerful changes in your body that support your energy, endurance, and overall health. These aren't just "fitness" benefits, they're practical adaptations that make a difference in how you feel and function day-to-day. No matter the stage of motherhood, all moms benefit from cardiovascular exercise; however, be sure to read the previous chapter for trimester trends and how they influence your body's adaptation to exercise. Let's examine these key benefits:

You Improve Your Stamina

- Cardio training increases both the number and efficiency of mitochondria, the energy-producing structures inside your cells. This means you're able to generate more energy to feel less drained from busy mom life.

- Aerobic exercise strengthens your heart, so it can pump more blood with each beat, a change known as increased stroke volume. It also strengthens your lungs and diaphragm. These changes mean you'll be less winded when carrying a sleeping child up the stairs or being convinced to roller skate with your nine-year-old.

- Your body also becomes better at using fat as a fuel source, especially during moderate or longer-duration activity, which means an afternoon walk instead of an additional cup of coffee may give you just the energy you need to get through witching hour.

- On top of that, aerobic exercise improves insulin sensitivity, helping your body regulate blood sugar more efficiently, which means fewer energy crashes and mood swings and better support for your long-term metabolic health.

You Keep Cool and Comfortable

- Dreading long summer days in an amusement park? Being aerobically fit means your body becomes better equipped to manage heat. You sweat more effectively, and blood flow to your skin increases so that you can cool yourself quicker.

The Mental Boost behind Aerobic Exercise

Aerobic exercise offers powerful mental health benefits. While research specific to mothers is still emerging, most experts agree that findings from the general population are applicable to pregnant and postpartum individuals. Before we dive into the benefits, it's worth reminding you that resistance training, or combining strength and cardio, can also support the emotional well-being described in this section.

- **Better Sleep:** You may not be in complete control over the amount of sleep you get, but I encourage you to do all that is in your power to improve the quality of sleep you get. Activities like brisk walking or light jogging can lead to better overall sleep quality. When done earlier in the day, it may help you fall asleep faster and wake up less often during the night. On the flip side, longer or more intense workouts (especially over ninety minutes in the evening) and too many high-intensity sessions in a week may disrupt sleep.[1]

- **Better Brain Function:** I wish more studies looked at how aerobic exercise impacts brain function during pregnancy, especially since so many women notice changes in memory and mental sharpness during this time. Still, we do know that cardio improves cognition (learning/understanding), memory (storing and retrieving information), and executive function (planning, organizing, controlling behavior) across all populations and ages[2] (another reason to be physically active with your kids!).

- **Better at Managing Stress:** How does feeling emotionally steady and ready to handle whatever motherhood throws at you sound? Well, evidence shows that aerobic exercise can help with that! Cardio supports your brain's ability to recover from stress and adjust to challenges. It also increases levels of BDNF (brain-derived neurotrophic factor), a protein that helps protect brain cells, support learning and memory, and buffer against the negative effects of stress.

- **Better Chance of Preventing or Managing Anxiety and Depression:** Regular aerobic activity is consistently linked to a lower risk of anxiety and depression. In one review, people who were more physically active had a 17 percent lower risk of depression and a 26 percent lower risk of anxiety compared to those who were less active. The researchers concluded that this relationship is probably causal, meaning it's not just a correlation; if you're inactive, your risk of developing anxiety and depression likely increases.[3]

How Much? How Often? How Hard?

As far as aerobic exercise recommendations, ACSM and CDC state: "All healthy adults aged 18–65 years should participate in moderate-intensity aerobic physical activity for a minimum of 30 minutes on five days per week, or vigorous-intensity aerobic activity for a minimum of 20 minutes on three days per week." Their recommendations during pregnancy and postpartum for moderate intensity are generally the same. Vigorous-intensity exercise is not part of the prenatal or postpartum exercise guidelines; however, the WHO states: "There was no reason to alter the amount or frequency of recommended moderate-intensity physical activity for pregnant and postpartum women compared with the general adult population. Women who, before pregnancy, habitually engaged in vigorous-intensity aerobic activity, or who were physically active, can continue these activities during pregnancy and the postpartum period."

Many wearable devices estimate your heart rate zones and will show when you're in the "moderate" or "cardio" range, typically between 64 and 76 percent of your max heart rate (calculated as 220 minus your age). You can also estimate moderate intensity by how you feel using the Modified Borg Scale, where on a scale of 0–10, 0 means no effort at all (like sitting or lying down) and 10 means maximum effort (the hardest exercise you can imagine). Moderate intensity typically falls in the 4–6 range. Lastly, the talk test is still a simple and effective tool; if you can talk but not sing, you're likely exercising at a moderate intensity.

It's also worth noting that while a lot of health advice focuses on how intense or frequent your workouts should be, there's growing evidence that just sitting too much can have its own risks, regardless of how much you exercise. According to the World Health Organization, spending too much time sitting or lying down (while awake) is linked to serious health issues like heart disease, certain cancers, type 2 diabetes, and even early death.

In other words, you can't completely "undo" hours of sitting with a single workout. Regular movement throughout the day, like walking, stretching, or just changing positions more often, really does matter. This is important to keep in mind if you're not able to stay active through pregnancy, or there is no time or energy for structured workouts after having a baby, or if you work a sedentary job.

Choosing Cardio

Now that you're familiar with the recommendations for aerobic exercise, the benefits, and how to choose the right intensity, it's time to explore which modality might work best for you. For many moms, this decision comes down to a combination of enjoyment, convenience, and selecting low or high impact. This section will help you thoughtfully select the type of aerobic activity to incorporate if cardiovascular fitness is a key focus.

High or Low Impact?

Every time you walk, run, or jump, your body absorbs force, especially through your bones and joints. That force is called impact. It's a common misconception that impact and intensity mean the same thing, but they don't. Impact is about how much force your body takes in when it hits the ground, while intensity describes how hard your body is working. Gravity plays a big role in impact by pulling you downward with each movement. Even walking involves some level of impact. Exercises are often categorized as low-impact or high-impact, depending on how your body moves during the activity.

- Low-impact exercises always keep at least one foot on the ground or eliminate ground contact altogether, like swimming or cycling.
- High-impact exercises, such as running or plyometrics, involve moments when both feet are off the ground. These activities can offer benefits like stronger bones, more resilient joints, and a faster increase in heart rate, but they also place more stress on the body.

The CFF method encourages you to begin with core training and function so that if you choose to progress to higher-impact activities, your strong, well-functioning muscles can serve as natural shock absorbers, helping to reduce the force placed on joints. By strengthening the core and surrounding muscle groups, you enhance your body's ability to distribute load and prevent excessive stress on any single joint, making high-impact activity safer and more sustainable.

You may be wondering whether high-impact activity is appropriate during pregnancy. The answer isn't one-size-fits-all. You can make an informed decision by reviewing the information in Chapters 4 and 5, paying attention to how your body feels during higher-impact movements and weighing the potential risks and benefits. Many moms choose to continue with more than just low-impact exercise, while others find high-impact activity uncomfortable, even outside of pregnancy. One approach isn't necessarily better than the other. The best choice is the one that feels right for you, your body, and your current needs. Let's take a look at two of the most common forms of aerobic exercise.

Walking for Moms

Everywhere you look, walking is recommended as the gold standard in aerobic fitness for health benefits. And although there is good reason for it (see benefits mentioned earlier), it still feels slightly boring to write about because we've heard it all before. However, as I think of how important walking has been in my journey, it isn't as bland. Here are a couple of ways walking has been useful to me:

Brain Boost

As I wrote this book, I'd get in the writing groove for a few hours and then my mind would start to drift, or I would feel my creativity lacking. Getting up for a short walk would get the ideas flowing again and buy me a couple more hours of productivity. Whether a lunchtime walk to get out of the office, a mile or two between client sessions, or a stroll to prevent writer's block, walking has always been a tool to boost my brain function.

Raising an Active Child

Looking back, I'm a little surprised I actually did this, but as soon as my daughter could walk, we often ditched the stroller. Living in a city, you often don't drive to get somewhere, or if you do, after you park, you still have a decent walk ahead of you. I honestly don't know how I had the patience to walk with a tiny-step two-year-old when I needed to be somewhere on time, but I did. I've always enjoyed walking places, and I wanted her to get used to it, too. Maybe she's just naturally that type of kid, or maybe it was the early start, but now, we walk everywhere together. She'll choose a brisk walk over a quick car ride to school any day.

Motivating Others

Walking (or wheeling) is one of the most universal and accessible forms of aerobic activity. It's a great entry point for people who aren't currently active, and sometimes, simply being out and visible can inspire someone else to take that first step. When my daughter was a newborn, walking while pushing her in a stroller was both my primary mode of transportation and my main form of exercise. We'd walk about 2.5 miles each way to attend a weekly baby group class. That's where I met Sybil, who lived at least a mile farther from the class than I did. One day, she asked if she could walk with me. I didn't think much of it at the time, but later she told me how I had inspired her to be more active.

I ended up training Sybil for over five years, and now she models an active lifestyle for her two daughters. She hasn't wavered in her commitment to fitness since. In no way am I taking credit for her active lifestyle; her level of dedication to anything she puts her mind to is truly inspiring, but it's one of my favorite postpartum walking memories, so I had to share.

Walking Considerations for Moms

- If you're using walking to meet the physical activity guidelines, you'll need to go beyond a casual stroll to reach moderate intensity. That means picking up the pace a bit. However, if your goal is simply to break up periods of inactivity, which also has meaningful health benefits, then, stroll away.

- If you live in a city with uneven sidewalks or lots of curbs, consider using a jogging stroller, even if you don't plan to run. They're generally easier to maneuver and have better suspension to keep your baby more comfortable. The downside? They tend to be bulkier and aren't as easy to bring in and out of the house.

- Although walking is a low-impact activity, supportive footwear still matters. What counts as "appropriate" can vary from person to person, but in general, your shoes should feel good during sustained movement and support your individual gait and needs.

- If you're babywearing while walking, tune into how your body feels, especially if you're still in the Core phase of CFF. Long walks with your baby on your chest can sometimes lead to back discomfort or trigger pelvic floor symptoms.

Running for Moms

It's funny because I've never called myself a runner, yet I've done plenty of running in my life. I've found many people either love it or hate it, and those who love it consider themselves runners, and those who hate it don't. I think I fall somewhere in between. I love it when it has a purpose, and for me, that purpose has varied.

In high school, I was on the track team and did the open 100 and 200, as well as the relays. Our school didn't have a proper track, so when we couldn't travel to another school's facilities, we'd run inside on cobblestone-like floors. That, without consistent strength training, was a recipe for disaster for me. I suffered chronic shin splints and even a stress fracture. Yet, I loved the feeling of competing, beating my personal records, and being on the team with my friends, so I kept running.

In college, I no longer ran track but eventually found my way back to running when I realized my eating and physical activity habits were not ideal. Only doing a few miles per week, I still didn't consider myself a runner. However, I realized that I no longer had issues with shin splints, and it was then that I identified the power of strength training. I had taken a semester course and became a regular in the gym. Stronger muscles meant better shock absorption and less injury for me. As an exercise science student, I was learning about all of the amazing ways your body adapts to exercise, so running was a way to live what I was learning.

After college, there was a 45-mile trail that ran behind my condo building. Most of my workouts took place in the multiple gyms where I worked, but running was convenient, so I maintained my casual running streak. I also discovered how caffeine can support endurance runs, so I started pushing for extra miles on occasion, and it didn't feel too bad being the sprinter I was.

Fast forward to pregnancy. At that time, I was living in Philadelphia. I didn't enjoy running through the neighborhoods, having to dodge people or pause at red lights, so I did most of my running workouts at the Temple University track, along the Schuylkill River path, or over the pedestrian lane on the Ben Franklin Bridge that connects Pennsylvania to New Jersey over the Delaware River. When I found out I was pregnant, I had to decide whether to keep running and maintain my sprint workouts. Because I didn't receive helpful advice, I dialed it back slightly in the first trimester due to uncertainty, but at some point, I realized it felt good to me and my body was handling it well, so I did my last pregnancy run at seven months with no negative effects to me or my daughter. In addition to craving the prenatal health benefits for both of us, running had always been a part of my life, so I think in some ways it helped me feel "normal" despite all of the changes my body was undergoing. And outside workouts on a nice day have always felt good to me, which was a feeling I wanted to maintain during pregnancy.

And how about this stage of life? Well, I still don't call myself a runner, but my daughter would classify me as one, which makes me feel great. She has memories from a very young age of her and me running together, and as soon as she started having her own running events, it came full circle, and she would ask me to join her on days when parents were invited to participate. Running also turned into a social activity and a way to connect with friends. Together we've done the Broad Street Run and the Philly 10K, which feel like must-dos if you're a "runner" in Philadelphia. Training for a race has also been a good way to raise money for a cause and remotivate myself with the training required. I've also used running to explore new cities I've visited.

Why did I share all of that? Because running has been a part of my life in different ways at different times, and I know that's true for a lot of moms. You don't have to be a runner, and you don't have to run. But if running is something you've loved, or something you're thinking about returning to after having a baby, whether recently or years ago, it's helpful to understand what that return might look like. Let's discuss the "return to running" guidelines and explore how running fits into the Core, Function and Fitness Approach.

Running through Motherhood

I was incredibly excited when the Postpartum Return to Running Guidelines came out. They do a fabulous job of guiding moms who want to return to running after having a baby. Because they're structured to be gradual and progressive, they complement the Core, Function and Fitness (CFF) approach well and can be used by any mom taking her first step toward running, no matter how long it's been since birth.

As for pregnancy, these guidelines can also serve as a helpful tool for evaluating whether running makes sense for you right now. For example, if you haven't been strength training or aren't able to perform some of the assessment exercises, you might decide that, given the added demands of pregnancy, running isn't the best fit for your current routine. If you're pregnant and you haven't been running or preparing your body for running, I personally don't see a good reason to start now or to set a postpartum running goal as your first step back into fitness.

Returning to Running Postnatal Guidelines

All of the guidance in this section has been pulled from the work of Tom Goom, Gráinne Donnelly, and Emma Brockwell, who made the information available to the public, to be informed and aware of important signs or symptoms that suggest a lack of readiness or reason to see a health professional.

Why a Gradual Approach Is Important

- Running is a high-impact activity that increases intra-abdominal pressure and stresses your recovering pelvic floor.

- Recovery of the pelvic floor and abdominal muscles improves four to six months after having a baby. By respecting this healing time, you'll reduce risks such as incontinence, pelvic organ prolapse, and diastasis recti.

- A step-by-step return ensures you enjoy the benefits of exercise while protecting your body as it heals.

How Do You Know If You're Ready?

The following exercises are good indicators that your strength and coordination have progressed. They're not meant to be a formal evaluation, but I share them because they offer a realistic picture of the movement control and strength that running demands, whether you're newly postpartum or years into motherhood. Understanding where you are now helps you make an informed decision about whether you're ready to gradually introduce running.

If you've worked through the Core and Function piece of my training approach, you've likely built a strong foundation and have set a goal to run because you've moved into the Fitness component. However, keep in mind that some of these movements, like the single-leg sit-to-stand or bounding, may require you to train them specifically to master them. Just because you can't perform one of them right now doesn't necessarily mean you're not capable or strong enough. It may simply mean your body hasn't practiced that particular skill yet. That's the principle of training specificity: to get better at a movement, you have to actually do it. With that said, here are the exercises that the three authors have identified as ones you should be able to do without pain, heaviness, dragging, or incontinence:

- Walk continuously for thirty minutes without discomfort.
- Hold a single-leg balance for at least ten seconds on each side.
- Twenty single-leg repetitions of exercises like calf raises, bridges, sit-to-stands, and side-lying leg abductions.
- Jog on the spot for one minute.
- Complete movements that require load transfer and balance, like forward bounds and hopping.

What Else Should You Consider before Running?

As we've touched on in other chapters, readiness for exercise isn't just about what your body can physically do. Below are a few additional factors to consider when deciding if you're ready to return to running.

- **Pelvic Health Assessment:** If possible, schedule an evaluation with a pelvic health physical therapist. They can assess for issues like urinary leakage, a noticeable gap in your abdominal wall, or sensations of heaviness, signs that may benefit from professional support before progressing to higher-impact exercise.
- **Psychological and Emotional Readiness:** Ask yourself why you want to return to running. Are you feeling internal or external pressure to do so? Have you been screened for postpartum depression or anxiety? Your mental and emotional health is just as important as your physical recovery.
- **Scar Mobilization:** If you've had a Cesarean birth or perineal tearing, gentle scar mobilization can support tissue healing and reduce stiffness. Some discomfort as you begin to move more

is normal, but it shouldn't feel like pain. If it does, check in with a healthcare provider.

- **Energy Management (RED-S):** Be mindful of Relative Energy Deficiency in Sport, a condition that can occur when your energy intake doesn't meet the demands of your activity. It can impact your recovery, bone health, menstrual cycle, and overall performance. Make sure you're fueling adequately to support both your movement and healing needs.

Wrapping It Up

You've learned how and why cardio fits into the fitness component of the Core, Function and Fitness approach. Although at the top of the pyramid, aerobic exercise, in addition to strength training, acts as an effective means to build endurance, support heart health, manage stress, and improve energy. Whether you choose low-impact movement or are ready to include higher-impact activities like running, the key accomplishment is twofold: advancing to this stage and identifying aerobic exercises that align with your needs.

Take Action

If you're moving on from Function to Fitness or ready to set aerobic fitness goals, choose one of the following to take the next step.

1. Assess whether your core is functioning well and whether you've built enough strength to support balance and absorb impact. If not, start with low-impact options while continuing to build strength through the Core and Function components of CFF.

2. Before resuming running or taking your first strides as a runner, review the foundational elements discussed in this chapter to assess your complete preparation, both mental resilience and physical capability, for this high-impact activity.

11

Putting It All Together

Key Insights from This Chapter

1. To develop your personalized exercise plan, you should determine and adapt how often you'll exercise, the intensity of your workouts, the type of exercise you're prioritizing, how long your sessions will be, and which phase of life you're in.
2. You shouldn't rely on willpower alone to stick with your exercise plan. Fitness professionals use evidence-based models to guide their clients and keep them on track, and you can use these same strategies to stay consistent with your plan.

As we near the end of the guide, I want to give you credit for taking the time to learn and understand not just about the value of exercise through all stages of motherhood but also how to make it work for you. We've covered all three components in the Core, Function and Fitness approach to mom fitness, and now it's time to bring it all together into a practical and personalized plan.

If you're not feeling thoughtful or creative right now, come back to this chapter at another time because it's that important. As I've done with hundreds of moms, I'll guide you through creating a fitness plan that fits your current life situation. This is a chapter you can revisit when your parenting season changes, when your children's routines alter your schedule, or as you reach your wellness goals. I'll share the same tips and strategies I've used with clients to help them stay active through pregnancy, recover stronger, and feel confident, energized, and capable in everyday life with their families.

As you're developing your plan, keep in mind that the intention is for you to be able to start using this plan tomorrow. This isn't a plan for next week or next month. This isn't an "ideal" plan or a plan that you picture yourself doing one day. This is a plan that is realistic for you now. The best exercise program is the one you can stick with, designed to fit your life, your challenges, and your goals. Most importantly, if you start putting your plan into action and find it hard to stay consistent, or realize your workouts are too easy, or maybe too ambitious, you can come back to this book, make some tweaks, and keep moving forward. This isn't all or nothing. It's not about perfection. This is your fitness journey through motherhood, meant to shift and evolve as you and your family do. Are you ready to begin?

Refresher

Let's start with a quick refresher in case it's been a while since you read the earlier chapters. Take a moment to revisit the self-assessment in Chapter 3. Why? Because having that reflection fresh in your mind will help guide the choices you make as you build your plan. I encourage you to jot down a quick summary of your key takeaways. What patterns or themes stood out? What factors do you need to keep in mind? And what's your overall impression of your current fitness needs, abilities, and reality?

Before you dive into the details of your plan, let's make sure it feels manageable. Instead of setting too many goals and falling short on all of them, choose your top one or two lifestyle priorities to support the fitness plan you're building. This helps you stay focused and increases your chances of following through. Here are sample priorities:

- Improve hydration.
- Improve nutrition.
- Improve quality (or amount) of sleep.
- See a healthcare professional or therapist for pain or symptoms that could interfere with physical activity.
- Reduce sedentary time with standing breaks, walking commutes, etc.
- Strategize how to overcome barriers like childcare, work, or fear.
- Maintain awareness of posture and positions that may cause muscle tightness or discomfort.

Now it's time to identify your starting point or where you currently fall within the CFF approach to mom fitness. While this isn't an exhaustive list, the following core focus areas can help you understand what to prioritize right now.

Core (Foundation)

- Achieve coordinated breathing and deep core activation.
- Learn to relax or contract pelvic floor muscles based on PT guidance.

- Stay consistent with foundational core exercises that target the essential core muscles (pelvic floor muscles, diaphragm, transverse abdominis, multifidus).
- Begin integrating core strength and stability into everyday movement and nontraditional core exercises.

Function (Middle Layer)

- Address pain or injuries with guidance from a physical therapist and stay consistent until you see progress.
- Master technique in all major "mom movement" patterns (squats, hinges, carries, pushes, pulls, and rotations/anti-rotation).
- Perform functional strength workouts consistently, meeting resistance training guidelines (at least 2x/week).
- Incorporate mobility exercises regularly to support strength, improve posture, and prevent compensation.

Fitness (Top of the Pyramid)

- Build on an established strength routine by adding variety, increasing challenge, or using more advanced training methods.
- Return to running or other high-impact activities following a gradual progression.
- If appropriate, work toward body composition or weight loss goals through training and nutrition.

You're now ready for the details of your plan as you should be clear on your personal needs, lifestyle priorities, and your starting point in CFF.

FITTT Principle

Let's start with a long-standing principle in the fitness industry known as FITT, which stands for Frequency, Intensity, Time, and Type. These four variables work together to shape the overall structure and effectiveness of your workouts. Frequency refers to how often you exercise. Intensity is how hard you're working during each session. Time is the length or duration of your workout. Type refers to the specific kind of activity you're doing, such as strength training, cardio, or flexibility work. When one of these elements changes, the others often need to adjust as well, making FITT a practical tool for customizing your plan and adapting it as needed.

You'll notice I've added an extra T to this section header. This stands for Trimester, which represents a three-month period. If you're pregnant or newly postpartum, this is an easy reference; each trimester naturally marks a distinct stage of change. But even beyond the fourth trimester, life with young kids tends to shift every few months. From dropping from two naps to one, or weaning from breastfeeding, their changing needs often reshape your schedule. And if your kids are older, "Trimester" can still apply; think of how different summer, with camps and vacations, feels compared to fall, with back-to-school routines and holidays. The point is, this extra T helps you consider the season of life you're in, making it a practical tool for planning a program that fits.

OK, get ready to take notes again, we're about to break down the FITTT principle. By the end of this section, you'll know how often you'll work out each week, at what intensity, for how long, and what type of exercise you'll be doing. Everything you decide here should connect back to what you've already reflected on earlier in this chapter.

We're going to walk through the FITTT variables in order, but you don't have to follow them that way when planning your workouts.

Since all five variables are interconnected, it often makes the most sense to start with the one that's either the most inflexible or most obvious to you. For example:

- If your daughter is on the travel soccer team and the next three months are going to be a bit chaotic with her sport and your new promotion at work, the Trimester you're in is pretty inflexible and the most relevant variable to identify first. You could also start with Time if you feel like the window of opportunity for workouts is your biggest barrier.
- If you're newly postpartum and beginning in the Core component of CFF, you could start with Type (core training) or Intensity (light to moderate), as those are a little clearer due to postpartum guidelines.

The key is to identify your anchor(s), the variable(s) that feel the most fixed or the easiest to decide right now, and build the rest of your plan around them. Let's revisit the first example: if you determine that you have fifteen minutes for each workout (Time) and you've identified functional strength training as your focus based on where you are in the Core, Function and Fitness framework, you already know two things: your Time is fifteen minutes, and your Type is strength training. If your current season feels like a busy "Trimester," that becomes a context-setting filter too.

From there, you'd adjust Frequency and Intensity to fit. That might mean working out five days a week with upper/lower body splits at a moderate intensity or doing full-body workouts in a circuit style to keep things efficient and focused on a bit higher intensity.

The point is: these choices aren't random. They're intentional. You're making each decision based on what fits your current reality, not forcing yourself into a plan that doesn't.

Before we break down each FITT variable, it's helpful to understand a few general patterns that can guide your decisions:

- Beginners often progress with less. If you're just starting (or restarting), lower frequency and intensity are not only enough, they're ideal. Your body is highly responsive to smaller amounts of movement.
- If you're training for something more advanced, like a race or performance-based goal, you'll likely need increased frequency, duration, and possibly intensity.
- Intensity affects recovery. The higher the intensity, the fewer sessions your body can recover from each week. On the flip side, low-to-moderate-intensity workouts can be done more often.
- Time impacts frequency. If your sessions are short (ten to fifteen minutes), you may be able to train more frequently. If they're longer (forty-five to sixty minutes), you might only manage a few focused sessions per week.
- Workouts don't need to have the same variables each session, and they probably won't. They can vary in time, type, and intensity to help you stay consistent, manage recovery, and fit movement into a changing schedule.

These are just general guidelines, not rules. Use them to help you adjust the other variables once you've identified your anchor.

Frequency: How Many Days per Week Will You Perform a Structured Exercise Session

Frequency refers to how many days per week you plan to engage in intentional movement or training. It's influenced by your goal, your schedule, your energy, and your ability to recover. It's important to be realistic here, even if your starting point is below the exercise guidelines. A two-day plan that you follow consistently is better than a four-day plan that never happens. Start with what's sustainable. How many days will you exercise?

Intensity: How Hard Will You Train? How Challenging Will Your Workouts Feel?

Intensity refers to the level of effort you put into a workout. Your intensity should reflect your current fitness level, your recovery capacity, and your primary goal. Lower intensity allows for more frequent training. Higher intensity requires more recovery and should be used more strategically. Remember, general exercise recommendations give you the flexibility to mix and match moderate intensity and moderate-vigorous intensity to meet your weekly minutes.

Time: How Long Will Each Exercise Session Be?

Time refers to the duration of each workout session, but I encourage you to also think of it as the Time of day. The duration might depend on your schedule, energy, and ability to stay consistent. The Time of day is similar but may also be influenced by when you have childcare or when you're least likely to be interrupted. Shorter workouts are often easier to fit into a busy day and may allow for more frequent training. Longer workouts might offer more volume or variety but often require more recovery and planning. Choose a session length you can stick with consistently, even during your busiest weeks. Most moms don't "find" time for exercise. You have to make it, and you should be purposeful about it. How much time will you set aside for each session?

Type: What Style of Exercise Will You Choose?

Type refers to the mode or style of exercise you're choosing, like strength training, walking, or core. This is often shaped by your stage in the Core, Function and Fitness framework, your goals, and what you have access to. This is also where my personal bias will show. If your frequency is one to two workouts per week, your Type should be core and/or strength training on both days. Choose your activity based on your goals. Not what's trendy, or what studio has the best New Year's deal, or because your sister-in-law got really great results with a specific app. Choose an activity that you're motivated to do and aligns with the frequency, intensity, type, time, and trimester you identify.

Another important factor in your selection is convenience. During the pandemic, we all switched to virtual workouts, and guess what, I saw a huge spike in progress and consistency in the moms I worked with. The convenience of not leaving your house and fitting in a workout between naps or meetings was so impactful that virtual sessions stayed on my menu of services and were a preference for many moms. What types of workouts will you do?

Trimester: What Will Life Look Like over the Next Three Months?

Trimester refers to the current season you're in, whether that's an actual trimester of pregnancy or simply a snapshot of your life right now. It's about understanding what external factors, like work, family schedules, travel, or energy levels, might influence how you train. This variable helps you frame realistic expectations and make sure your plan fits within your actual capacity, not just your intentions.

If you do happen to be pregnant, consider how some of the pregnancy trends we discussed will interact with these variables. Are you feeling fearful about exercise? If so, choose a Type of exercise that is familiar and that you're comfortable with, even if it isn't completely aligned with your goals. The same goes for frequency. Start with one day per week until you're ready to add more. What's coming up in the next three months that might impact your routine?

FITTT Moms

To further illustrate the principles of FITTT, I'll provide you with a few examples from moms I've worked with. I'll walk you through the summary of their personal assessment, stage of CFF, and how they structured their exercise plan based on the interacting variables.

Alexis

Alexis has two kids, ages three and six. She chose to prioritize nutrition to support her new exercise plan. She has a strong fitness foundation and categorizes herself in the Fitness component.

- **Frequency:** Although she's an experienced exerciser, she's identified three days per week as the most realistic for her.
- **Intensity:** Her core is strong, and she's been strength training consistently for months. Although it's safe for her to choose vigorous intensity, she doesn't enjoy it. She opts for moderate-intensity exercise for each workout.
- **Time:** All her workouts are going to be completed with a personal trainer or group in exercise classes, so the duration of her workouts will range from forty-five to sixty minutes.
- **Type:** She spent months mastering mom movements and is loving how she feels, so she wants to keep prioritizing strength

training for all three workouts. She plans to stay active outside of structured sessions by walking her kids to school every day.

- **Trimester:** She just started a new job, so she's in a work-committed trimester. She decides to do all early morning sessions so that nothing can get in her way and she can spend the evening with her family.

Kelly

Kelly is pregnant with twins, and at thirteen weeks pregnant, she is feeling pretty good. She is a casual runner and yoga enthusiast. She has an extremely busy job, and it keeps her on her feet all day. Sometimes she's so busy that she doesn't eat or drink enough, so she chooses to prioritize drinking more water and afternoon snacks to better support her fitness plan and pregnancy. Because she knows her body will change rapidly with twins, she takes a step back from the prepregnancy Fitness category she was in and commits to Function as her primary goal.

- **Frequency:** She was working out five days per week, but she's taken on more shifts before going on maternity leave. Because of this, she dials it back to three times per week.
- **Intensity:** She has no contraindications and plans to stick with moderate-intensity exercise. However, on days when she is tired from long days at work, she will regress to low-intensity physical activity.
- **Time:** Given she dropped from five days to three, she has increased her frequency from thirty minutes to forty minutes to feel like she is maintaining her training volume for as long as she can.

- **Type:** This variable will change depending on her work schedule. If her day starts in the afternoon, she will go on morning runs. Running provides a huge mental benefit to her, and she hasn't experienced any pelvic floor symptoms, so she is choosing to continue unless it becomes uncomfortable. If she starts work early in the morning, she will take a restorative prenatal yoga class after work. She also plans to do one full-body strength training session each week, two if her schedule allows, as she knows that's ideal.
- **Trimester:** She's in her second trimester, so she has pretty good energy and is still moving well, so no major modifications are needed. However, she does want to be more intentional about breathing and deep core activation.

Sydney

Sydney has an eight-week-old baby. She's never had a consistent fitness routine, but she's feeling weak and finding it difficult to move through her day comfortably. Sydney falls into the Core layer of the CFF pyramid. She has identified her lifestyle priority to be seeing a physical therapist for an evaluation and instruction on how to massage her C-section scar.

- **Frequency:** Exercise is new to her, but because her duration is going to be low and she'll benefit from more frequent mobility and core sessions, she sets her frequency to three days per week.
- **Intensity:** She's still moving rather slowly and recovering after the C-section, so her workouts will be low-intensity.
- **Time:** Her sessions will average ten to fifteen minutes for two of her workouts and will see a postpartum exercise specialist for a thirty-minute session on her third workout.

- **Type:** Given her focus on healing and core, her shorter workouts will be targeted core sessions focused on coordinating deep core activation and breath. Her longer session with her trainer will additionally include mobility exercises.
- **Trimester:** She's in the fourth trimester, so she is giving herself grace by balancing rest and physical activity. If she's had several days without sleep, she'll plan to complete her short workouts at the first opportunity in the morning so that she can prioritize rest later in the day. Her partner agreed to stay with the baby on the days she goes to her personal training session or physical therapy.

Complete Your Plan

You'll notice that we didn't get into specific exercise selection or detailed workout plans, and that is intentional. This entire guide is about personalizing and adapting workouts for your specific needs, and with the information in this book, you'll now be able to do that. Not only are you empowered to select or create workouts, but you have the knowledge to progress and regress them as needed so that you can stay consistent and see results. Some of you will feel motivated to design workouts on your own, and others will choose to identify online programs or find a boutique studio that aligns with your FITT plan. Here is how it works:

- If you're selecting your own exercises, you can refer back to the chapters on core, functional strength training, and fitness or cardio that align with your objectives. You can use the exercise examples provided in those chapters or explore the resources named in the appendix, or you can search for new ideas that meet your needs. For example, you can use search terms or prompts like, "I am returning to exercise and need a list of push pattern exercises. They should be moderate skill and intensity and require no equipment. Act like a maternal exercise specialist and provide a bulleted list in a progressive sequence from least challenging to most." You could do this for each movement pattern, to build the workout that fits into your plan.

- For those of you planning to follow a program online or attend classes at your gym, use your FITT plan to guide strategic choices and avoid hopping between random workouts that don't align with your desired outcomes. For example, if your plan includes two thirty-minute moderate-intensity sessions, shifting your priority from core training to overall functional strength, you'd avoid "booty burn" or "arms and shoulders" and instead look for full-body strength programs that primarily train the major movement patterns.

- If you plan to work with a personal trainer, they should be qualified to plan your sessions without much input from you; however, don't let it be a passive process. Use your plan to identify what you need your trainer's guidance for and to ensure you're selecting a trainer that is aligned with your priorities. For example, if you just set a Fitness goal to run a 5K, maybe you're following a "couch to 5K" training plan, but you need a trainer to support your strength training sessions so that you're focusing on muscles and movements to help prevent injury.

Beyond Willpower

Now that you've created your plan, let's talk about starting and sticking with it. Maintaining an exercise routine isn't just about willpower, and behavior change doesn't happen overnight. It's a process shaped by your mindset, environment, and readiness. Fitness professionals use evidence-based models to guide clients through this process, and you can use those same strategies to set yourself up for success. These models can help you better understand your own patterns and identify what will help you follow through.

You've probably experienced pieces of each model as you've made changes or reached goals in the past. Don't overthink it, skim through and go with the one that resonates most or reflects how you've successfully created change before.

Social Cognitive Theory (Learning from Others and Yourself)

This theory explains that we learn behaviors by watching others, by thinking about our environment, and by believing in our own ability (self-efficacy) to succeed. For example, if you're on a group all-inclusive vacation and one of your friends goes to Aqua Aerobics at the pool every morning while her husband has breakfast with the kids, you might feel confident that you can do it too. The environment makes it possible, your friend has shown you it's doable, and you feel you're fit enough for a leisurely pool workout, so you adopt the behavior and join her.

Think about behaviors you've successfully changed in the past. Did someone inspire or teach you, making it easier to get started? Did your environment, like a supportive community, help set you up for success? Did you feel confident in your ability to make the change? If this resonates with you, the following strategies could help:

- Start with a manageable plan that you feel confident you can follow. Focus on technique and mastering skills before progressing.
- Set up your home workout space for success and have your equipment ready before each session.
- Remember, you're now part of the Active Mom community, and hundreds of other moms are using exercise as a tool. Surround yourself with others on a similar path.

Health Belief Model (Weighing Risks and Benefits)

This theory suggests that people change their behavior if they believe they're at risk for a serious health problem, think the issue is severe, feel the benefits of action outweigh the barriers, and have the confidence to act. For example, if you learn heart disease runs in your family, and understand exercise can help, and believe you're capable of daily walks, you might start going on family strolls every night after dinner.

Think about the times you've made changes for your health. Were you motivated by wanting to prevent future health issues? Did understanding the benefits make it easier to act? Did you weigh the effort required against the potential rewards? If so:

- Continue to remind yourself of all the ways exercise positively impacts your health, like managing postpartum depression or reducing your risk of cancer.
- Keep track of improvements in your daily life, like getting to the end of the day without having lower back pain.

- Reread the empowering information in this book to keep your health and wellness at the front of your mind.

Social-Ecological Model (Layers of Influence on Our Choices)

This model recognizes that successful change depends on support at different levels, from your personal choices to your family dynamics to your community resources. For example, you might begin a prenatal fitness class because you personally want to feel strong during pregnancy, your OB/GYN supports it, your neighborhood gym offers it, and maternal health policies encourage physical activity during pregnancy.

Reflect on changes you've maintained long term. Did having support from family or friends make a difference? Did changing your surroundings help change your habits? If this connects with you, consider these approaches:

- Involve your family in creating a schedule that supports your workout time and put it on a shared calendar.
- Find ways to be physically active with your family, doing things that everyone enjoys.
- Connect with local resources like pre/postnatal personal trainers, stroller-friendly walking groups, or when spending time with friends, choose a fitness class over dinner.
- Use the CFF approach and this guide as a supportive resource.

When I was postpartum, this model influenced many moms who were a part of the baby group I was in. One of the moms proposed that in addition to our weekly child-focused class, we bring our babies to a postpartum yoga class. There was a studio in the area that was willing to do a private class once per week just for our group. The camaraderie from the group, the resources within our community, the choice we were all making to take care of ourselves postpartum, all led to a consistent exercise routine.

Transtheoretical Model of Change (Stages of Changing Habits)

This theory says people go through stages when adopting healthier habits, such as thinking about change, preparing, taking action, and maintaining it. For instance, you might start by just thinking about getting back into swimming (contemplation), then you start researching pool schedules (preparation), then you attend an open swim (action), and eventually you have a pool membership and you're going once per week (maintenance).

Think about times you've adopted a healthier behavior. Did you need time to prepare and plan? Did planning small steps make it easier to begin? If this sounds familiar, try these strategies:

- Honor your current stage of readiness and skip the "I should do" mentality.
- Don't skip planning. Be deliberate on how you'll get from "thinking about" exercise to "maintaining" a consistent program.
- Follow the CFF method and start where you are, progressing step by step.

Theory of Planned Behavior (Intentions Shape Our Actions)

This theory focuses on how strong intentions turn into actions. It suggests that your attitude about exercise, what others think, and your confidence all shape your commitment to follow through on your plans. For example, if you are excited about starting your personal training sessions, your family thinks it's important, and you feel capable of fitting it into your schedule, you'll likely stick to the plan.

Think about the changes you've made that started with a strong intention. What was your attitude toward the change? Did you feel it was more beneficial than burdensome? Did you feel encouragement from family, friends, rather than pressure to make the change? How much control did you feel you had over your ability to make and maintain the change? If this resonates with you, these strategies may help:

- Examine your true feelings about the type of exercise you choose. Start with forms of movement you enjoy.

- Consider whose opinions influence your exercise decisions and build a supportive network. Share your fitness goals with a supportive friend, family member, or accountability partner.

- Celebrate your wins, like booking a class and making it there on time, signing up for a 5K and finishing, or getting successfully discharged from physical therapy.

I can think of a few moms whom I've worked with who have benefited from these strategies. One mom comes to mind, as during her pregnancy she was very open about the fact that she never stayed consistent in the past with exercise because she doesn't enjoy it. Knowing her attitude could be a barrier to her having an active pregnancy, she signed up for sessions with me. Additionally, her husband provided the support she needed by walking her to her session each week. With these strategies, she was able to stay active and celebrate how exercise played a role in improving her mental health during pregnancy and improved her feelings about exercise overall.

Practical Solutions

Hopefully, you were able to relate to one of those models and gather a couple of strategies. Knowing barriers that moms specifically may face, this last section of the chapter will provide you with a few additional ways to prevent and overcome barriers so that you can succeed in the plan you developed. If they align well with a particular behavior change model, I've mentioned it, but most of these can tie to several models and are relevant for most moms and moms-to-be.

Involve Your Children

Research shows a strong link between the physical activity levels of parents and their children. Specifically, there is a direct, positive association between the amount of physical activity a mother engages in and how active her child is. When moms move more, their kids tend to follow suit.[1] By modeling an active lifestyle, parents play a crucial role in developing healthy movement habits early in life, which can have lasting benefits for their children's health and well-being.

So, what does this look like in practice? I'll give a snapshot of my personal journey, which I've also seen mimicked in my clients. When my daughter was a newborn and I was returning to fitness, I'd prop her on a breastfeeding pillow on the mat next to me. I'd distract her and keep her happy throughout my short workouts. When I progressed to running, she joined me in the jogging stroller, and when she was able to walk, I'd take her to the track where I could keep an eye on her in the infield as I did sprints. When she was around four, I started the habit of Saturday morning home workouts. And what did my efforts lead to besides my ability to stay consistent with physical activity? Eventually, during the track workouts, she would join me, yes, even at age three. During Saturday morning workouts, she began to play with the colorful bands and then eventually asked to join me and would even call me out if I didn't start my day with exercise. Now, she still enjoys screen time, but she is naturally active, and it's just a part of her life and mine.

From a behavior change standpoint, working out with or in front of your kids taps into several of the models we reviewed.

- According to Social Cognitive Theory, children learn through observation. When they consistently see you moving your body, they internalize that behavior as part of what's normal.
- The Health Belief Model also comes into play here. When moms recognize the long-term health benefits for both them and their children, it becomes easier to justify the effort.
- The Social-Ecological Model reminds us that the home environment matters. Your household is its own little ecosystem, and home workout routines establish a norm of physical activity.

Working out with children can feel messy and inconvenient at first, but those small efforts add up, and it does get easier. When movement is shared with your kids, it becomes a family value. This can help you stay consistent with your FITT plan, regardless of which model it's tied to.

Scheduling Workouts

Whether a wall calendar or in your phone, if you are someone who lives by a schedule and calendar, then booking your workouts just like appointments is the tool for you. Just like you wouldn't miss a doctor's visit or parent-teacher conference, your workouts deserve the same priority. Take a few moments each week to plan ahead. Pull up your calendar and block out specific times for your workouts. Write them down or set reminders and commit to showing up for yourself. When life happens and you don't have a choice but to miss the workout, take the extra step in rescheduling it. Don't get to Friday realizing you only hit one of your three workouts because you didn't hold yourself accountable. Set the tone for yourself, your family, and your coworkers that exercise is nonnegotiable.

- The Theory of Planned Behavior is supported in this strategy by reinforcing a clear intention and having a sense of control, knowing when you'll exercise.
- From a Social-Ecological Model perspective, treating workouts as nonnegotiable appointments can help shape family and community expectations so that everyone understands and supports your exercise routine as part of the weekly structure.

Treating your workouts like any other appointment, and protecting those time slots, encourages consistent follow-through, making it more likely you'll stick to FITTT.

Top Five Priorities

I'm sure you are constantly managing competing priorities, and it's easy for exercise to get sidelined. Creating a "top five" list each week helps you focus on what truly matters and provides you with an opportunity to regularly revisit the benefits and barriers of exercise. If you're a to-do list mama, this tool is for you. If work is a priority, define exactly what's most important (preparing a report, responding to urgent emails, submitting expenses), identifying specific tasks is better than being vague and prioritizing everything about work. If family time is on your top five list, again, be specific. Knowing you may not be able to "do it all," decide whether it's quality time at the park or doing bedtime routines. The clearer you are, the easier it is to focus. Understand that your list will change weekly, or even daily. Some weeks, fitness might top the list; other weeks, it may take a backseat to deadlines or family events. If your FITTT plan is in your top five, let less critical tasks wait. For example, if walking makes your list, emails or cleaning can come after your workout. If fitness doesn't make the list, that's okay, use this strategy to make peace with what you can accomplish without guilt. This approach keeps you focused on what matters, helping you stay accountable without feeling overwhelmed.

- This strategy bolsters commitment through the Health Belief Model, by explicitly recognizing the benefits of working out and actively reducing barriers by placing fitness high on your list.
- The list approach also reflects Social Cognitive Theory because prioritizing movement is a form of self-regulation, you're consciously managing day-to-day decisions based on what you value most.

By specifying which activities matter most right now, you can increase the likelihood that you'll follow through on the goals you set.

Build a Support System and Overcome Mom Guilt

You don't think twice about enlisting professionals to help with taxes or getting a haircut, or getting a babysitter for a date night, yet when it comes to fitness, guilt often sneaks in. The term "mom guilt" exists for a reason. Moms tend to put their needs last, viewing exercise as a luxury rather than an essential part of their well-being. Many feel guilty when taking time away from their kids, investing money in a gym or trainer, or asking for childcare support. It's a bit funny when you think about it, because during pregnancy, moms-to-be make healthy decisions all the time for the benefit of the baby, but as soon as the baby is born, taking care of yourself for the benefit of your child isn't as obvious or intuitive.

Building a support system so that you can maintain your fitness plan without mom guilt isn't selfish. This might look like buying a package with a personal trainer or finding a babysitter. If the support you're seeking comes from friends or family, you should start by being clear about your needs. Do you need childcare for sixty minutes per week? Do you need a workout buddy for the remainder of your third trimester? Let them know specifically how they can support you. You may find it beneficial to set a recurring schedule so that you're not having the conversation each week, and it just becomes routine.

- When moms actively seek childcare help, join mom-focused fitness groups, or hire a trainer, it can foster lasting change through the Social-Ecological Model by involving multiple layers of support.

- This also ties into the Theory of Planned Behavior, because having a supportive circle reshapes subjective norms (exercise is being encouraged, not selfish).

- Finally, Social Cognitive Theory is evident as moms witness positive outcomes (more energy, better mood) and strengthen their belief that prioritizing fitness benefits the whole family, helping to counteract any guilt.

Adapt during Transitions

One of the best pieces of advice I received at my baby shower was to remember that parenting is a culmination of stages and phases for both me and my child (thanks, Dione!). This advice was intended to reassure me that challenging times were just a stage and to take the time to enjoy the positives of each phase. This piece of advice is one to keep front and center as you aim to stay consistent with your FITTT plan. Whether it's returning to work after maternity leave or your child's sleep regression, these transitions and changes require you to be adaptable.

During a transition or period of change, start by acknowledging that the schedule or routine you previously committed to might not be the best for this stage. As you figure out this new stage, perhaps plan to maintain your exercise routine rather than progress. This might mean choosing just a few exercises to sprinkle in throughout the day or opting for home workouts instead of the gym until you can adjust to the new schedule. Give yourself grace and time to figure out what works for you as you transition to a new phase, aiming for maintenance and not perfection while you get settled.

- Being adaptable may boost your confidence that you can handle new challenges, and we know that self-efficacy plays a major role in the Social Cognitive Theory.
- From a Social-Ecological Model standpoint, acknowledging that phases change and seeking flexible routines also underscores how personal behavior is influenced by the evolving dynamics of family and community demands, ensuring workouts remain feasible regardless of life's ups and downs.

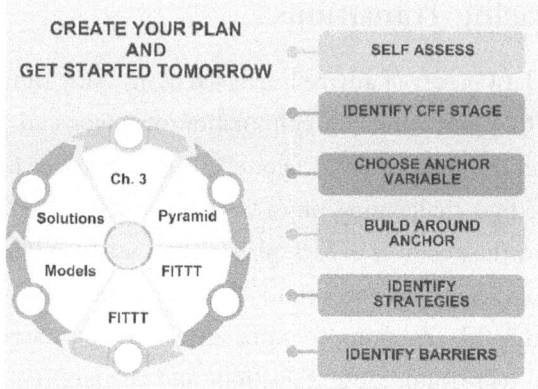

Develop your plan. A summary of the steps outlined in this chapter. It's a continuous, cyclical process as your life goes through changes and as you meet fitness goals. Created by author in Canva; © Ashley Reid.

You now have a road map to build sustainable habits using the FITTT principle and behavior change strategies. By focusing on small, consistent actions and adjusting your approach as life changes, you can create a fitness routine that not only supports your health but also sets a lasting example for your family. Please refer to this chapter if you're finding it difficult to follow your plan or when you're ready for a new one.

Take Action

> This is the last chapter! Whether you've been reading this guide over time, finished it in one sitting, or this is your tenth time returning to it, I applaud your commitment to nurturing both your emotional and physical strength. You deserve to feel fit, strong, and confident as you move through motherhood! Below you'll find the two next steps to choose from just like the other chapters, but with this being the last chapter, I've also included my final call to action. Thanks for trusting me, and I'm glad that you're part of the Active Mom community!

Chapter 11 Options

1. Go back to Chapter 3 and reflect on your current needs, barriers, and goals. Update your notes and identify one to two lifestyle priorities to focus on right now.

2. Using the FITTT principle, outline a realistic and actionable exercise plan. Focus on what's doable now, not ideal someday.

Final Call to Action

You've put in the time, done the work, and hopefully challenged a few assumptions along the way. As you move forward, remember, you're not just doing this for yourself, you're doing it with others, as part of a bigger shift in how we approach the sport of motherhood.

1. Let your efforts be visible. When you make choices that prioritize your strength and well-being, others notice. You become part of the change simply by showing up, speaking honestly, and supporting others doing the same.

2. Lean on your people and be there for them too. Whether it's your partner, a friend, or someone in the Active Mom community, give and receive support. We weren't meant to navigate this alone.

3. Advocate for the care you deserve. Use what you've learned to ask better questions, speak up about what's missing, and clearly communicate your needs, whether you're working with a healthcare provider, a pelvic floor PT, or a fitness professional. Exercise is just one part of the picture, but it can be a powerful entry point for change.

4. Stay tuned in and curious. Block out the noise that sells shame or bounce-back culture. Keep learning from sources rooted in evidence, not pressure.

5. Keep using the Core, Function and Fitness method, because it's designed for moms just like you (see Appendix A for a slightly more personal closing to this book, a letter to you).

Appendix A
My Letters to You

I hope that while reading this book, you've felt my genuine belief that all moms can find a way to make exercise work for them, and that you deserve support from someone who truly understands your needs. These personal letters are an extension of that support, offering encouragement and insights that didn't fit in the main chapters but may be exactly what you need right now. You'll find a few included here. For more letters and additional resources, visit www.activemomfitness.com.

Dear New Mom,

First, let's celebrate you! The early days of motherhood are filled with so many emotions and new experiences. Because you're reading this letter, it tells me you're doing your best, and that's not always easy, so I applaud you and welcome you to the Active Mom community.

From sleepless nights to physical recovery, you're managing a lot, and the thought of exercise can feel daunting. If you're experiencing the baby blues or facing anxiety or depression, that adds another layer of complexity. We're often expected to immediately exude gratitude and joy but know that you are not alone if you're struggling to connect with your baby or your new identity as a mom.

It might be hard to see beyond today's challenges, but every mom I've worked with began with the foundational steps of Core, Function and Fitness was able to see progress and move forward. Picture a future where you feel stronger, more energized, and more confident in your body. A day where you have the stamina to chase your toddler, the strength to carry your child without strain, and the mental clarity to handle life's demands with resilience. It starts with believing that even small actions will help you be the mom you want to be.

At this stage, healing and recovery are your top priorities. That might mean doing a few mobility exercises (especially for your chest and upper back) after the morning feed, seeing a physical therapist for postpartum concerns, scheduling an appointment to address mental health, or simply figuring out how to fit nourishing snacks into your day. Don't overwhelm yourself by thinking beyond your starting point. The place you've reached today matters and is sufficient.

Lastly, I ask that you please tune out the bounce-back culture and try to connect with moms who can relate to you. You can find a mom tribe in your community or online. Avoid following influencers on social media who make you feel bad about your path and your return to physical activity. I assure you that one day soon, you'll wake up feeling a little more like yourself.

Former new mom,
Ashley

Dear C-Section Mom,

How are you feeling? As I'm writing to you, I'm wondering if your C-section was planned and it went well or was it an emergency and a traumatic experience? In either case, if it wasn't the way you'd hoped your birth would go, I'm sorry and hope you get a chance to share your story.

I also wonder if you're able to prioritize your healing and recovery while taking care of a newborn. I distinctly remember being in the hospital and feeling determined to go down to the next floor where my daughter was, so I could breastfeed her at 3 a.m. Because of the pain from my C-section, it took me ten minutes just to get out of my room, and by the time I made it down to her, they had already fed her. I was devastated and felt the weight of failure. The point is that Cesareans are major surgeries and can have serious implications. I hope you're able to give yourself some grace and that you have someone reassuring you that your needs matter too.

I'd also remind you that initial healing can take weeks to months, but that rebuilding your strength and addressing core stability can take upward of a year. The Core, Function and Fitness approach is there to support you, but remember you're permitted to move at your own pace. If you're fortunate to be feeling good, you still want to follow a gradual progression, so your tissues can continue to heal.

As you resume activity, you may notice numbness, pulling sensations around your scar, and discomfort in your abdomen. These are common experiences caused by how the surgery affects the nerves in your lower abdomen and the scar tissue that forms as you heal. Be sure to ask your doctor at your checkup appointment if you're ready for scar tissue massage and how to do it. This is a simple task that improves blood flow and prevents adhesion. However, I've worked with many moms who couldn't bring themselves to touch or even look at the scar. This is a normal response. If you're unable to do it, ask your partner or see a physical therapist. If you begin scar tissue massage and there are any signs of redness, swelling, or discharge, please go back to your doctor. If you'd describe the pulling in your abdomen as you return to exercise as "discomfort," this is also normal, but the feeling shouldn't be described as "pain" or linger after the workout.

I'll end with stating that your body is remarkable, and it knows how to heal. Please just ensure you're creating a healing environment by staying hydrated, consuming adequate nutrients, and progressively returning to physical activity. You have the same ability as moms who delivered vaginally to reach your fitness potential.

Fellow C-section Mom,
Ashley

Dear Mom, in Pelvic Floor Physical Therapy,

   I feel like I should start simple and say, yes, it's worth it! You've chosen to invest in yourself, and that's something to be proud of, especially when it feels like there's so much else competing for your time and energy. I know this journey can be frustrating, physically and emotionally. Pelvic floor issues can affect everything from how you care for your child to your relationship with your partner, and it's normal to feel at a loss or even blindsided by a condition you may not have expected. I remember learning about hypertonic pelvic floor issues not through my exercise science textbooks or birth preparation but through personal postpartum experience. Like many moms, I wasn't expecting it and discovering it firsthand while also healing from a C-section was difficult.

   And then there's the PT "homework" you're supposed to do between sessions, while you're relaxed, and probably alone (for the internal work). It's so easy to feel like you're failing when you find it impossible to find the time and mindset to be consistent with these exercises. Even though these exercises may seem minimal compared to other fitness routines, they can feel like a massive effort when you're transitioning to a new routine and family dynamics, while also coping with a lack of energy.

   Here's what I want you to know: although frustrating now, PT is also an opportunity. By working with your physical therapist, you're building a stronger core, a fitness foundation, and better movement patterns that have a long-lasting impact on both your quality of life and future workouts. Focusing so specifically on muscle groups that don't usually get enough attention is a gift, even though it won't feel like that now.

   I'm pleased that the stigma around pelvic floor issues is fading, and we're able to talk about it openly. Because of this, effective treatments are more widely available. You're not alone, there is support, and you're not stuck. Progress may take time, but it's possible, and every small step forward is worth it.

This book is unique because it was written with moms like you in mind, from the perspective of someone who's been through pelvic floor therapy, has collaborated with expert physical therapists, and has helped countless moms as they rebuild their relationship with fitness during and after treatment. Use this book as a resource, whether you're in the thick of therapy or transitioning to your next fitness goals. Share it with your physical therapist to ensure that your exercises and treatment plan align seamlessly.

You're already doing the hard work by showing up for yourself. Stay consistent with your therapy, and don't be afraid to lean on the support available to you. Healing isn't always linear, but progress is possible. Keep going, and trust that there's a stronger, more confident version of you waiting on the other side.

With encouragement and understanding,
Ashley

To the Mom Who Feels Guilty Taking Time to Exercise,

Whether consciously or somewhere in the fabric of your being, the need, pressure, or expectation to put other people's needs before your own is a commonly known mom trait. So, it's no wonder that carving out time for yourself can feel like you're neglecting something, or someone. In this letter, I'm going to gently challenge that guilt, while also acknowledging that mom guilt is common and not just a switch that can be turned off.

For me personally, I realized that when others care for my daughter, she benefits from experiencing the love and attention from someone besides me. If I were working out at home and had to tell her that mommy is busy, I looked at it as an opportunity for her to be creative and learn ways to entertain herself. Additionally, I always felt like I was showing her how to value her own needs and how to keep healthy habits a priority.

For many of the moms I worked with, exercise became nonnegotiable after they saw the mental and emotional benefits and the positive impact it had on their relationship with their family. Exercise can help reduce stress, anxiety, and depression, and they would notice the difference in how they felt and how they parented when they became inconsistent in their routine.

I encourage you to reframe how you think of exercise, so you can reduce the feelings of guilt. Consider exercise as more than just movement, it's an investment that pays dividends in your ability to play energetically with your kids after a long day, develop the physical capability to do things like ice skate or play catch, demonstrate healthy priorities, and ultimately influence your children's lifelong relationship with fitness.

That guilt you feel. It's temporary. When exercise becomes part of your family's routine, those feelings will fade, replaced by pride in creating a healthier environment for everyone. Shift your mindset to think of exercise not as competing with your role as a mom but as an essential part of it.

With encouragement,
Ashley

Appendix B
Additional Resources

Stay in touch with Ashley Reid

- Instagram: @activemomfitness
- LinkedIn: @ashleyreidexphys
- YouTube: @ashleyreidexphys
- www.activemomfitness.com

This is a QR code that will take readers to Active Mom Fitness to explore resources and the blog. Created by author in Canva; © Ashley Reid.

Visit https://www.corefunctionfitness.com/.

Appendix B 241

This is a QR code that will take readers to Core, Function and Fitness resources to explore. Created by author in Canva; © Ashley Reid.

- Free CFF courses and programs
- Video demonstrations and sample workouts-movement patterns, working around the pelvis
- Downloadable personal self-assessment
- Step-by-Step Programs—Mom Butt, Best for the Bump, Core Foundation Series, Transitioning from Pelvic Floor PT to Exercise and more!

Continuing Education Courses for Fitness Professionals (https://www.acefitness.org/)

Appendix B

This is a QR code that will take fitness professionals to related continuing education courses. Created by author in Canva; © Ashley Reid.

Search for:

- Effective Pre/Postnatal Client Assessment Strategies
- Core Training Essentials for Pregnancy and Postpartum

The Canadian Society for Exercise Physiology (https://csep.ca/category/publications/get-active-questionnaire/)

- Get Active Questionnaire Pregnancy
- Get Active Questionnaire Postpartum

Maternal Mental Health Resources

- Postpartum Support International (PSI) (https://postpartum.net/)
- Maternal and Child Health Bureau (MCHB) (https://mchb.hrsa.gov/)
- Perinatal Mental Health Tool Kit (https://www.acog.org/programs/perinatal-mental-health)

Notes

Introduction

1 "Postpartum," *Merriam-Webster*, https://www.merriam-webster.com/dictionary/postpartum (accessed April 13, 2025).

Chapter 2

1 A. Bryndal, M. Majchrzycki, A. Grochulska, S. Glowinski, and A. Seremak-Mrozikiewicz, "Risk Factors Associated with Low Back Pain among a Group of 1510 Pregnant Women," *Journal of Personalized Medicine* 10, no. 2 (2020): 51, https://doi.org/10.3390/jpm10020051.

2 Okafor, Uchenna Benedine, and Daniel Ter Goon, "Physical Activity Advice and Counselling by Healthcare Providers: A Scoping Review," *Healthcare* 9, no. 5 (2021): 609, https://doi.org/10.3390/healthcare9050609.

3 World Health Organization, *Guidelines on Physical Activity and Sedentary Behaviour* (Geneva: World Health Organization, 2020), https://www.who.int/publications/i/item/9789240015128 (accessed April 13, 2025).

4 L. Zhou, X. Feng, R. Zheng, Y. Wang, M. Sun, and Y. Liu, "The Correlation between Pregnancy-Related Low Back Pain and Physical Fitness Evaluated by an Index System of Maternal Physical Fitness Test," *PLoS ONE* 18, no. 12 (2023): e0294781, https://doi.org/10.1371/journal.pone.0294781.

5 C. Duchette, M. Perera, S. Arnett, E. White, E. Belcher, and R. Tinius, "Benefits of Resistance Training during Pregnancy for Maternal and Fetal Health: A Brief Overview," *International Journal of Women's Health* 16 (2024): 1137–47, https://doi.org/10.2147/IJWH.S462591.

6   C. T. Miller, S. F. Fraser, I. Levinger, N. E. Straznicky, J. B. Dixon, J. Reynolds, and S. E. Selig, "The Effects of Exercise Training in Addition to Energy Restriction on Functional Capacities and Body Composition in Obese Adults during Weight Loss: A Systematic Review," *PLoS ONE* 8, no. 11 (2013): e81692, https://doi.org/10.1371/journal.pone.0081692.

7   L. Ferla, C. Darski, L. L. Paiva, G. Sbruzzi, and A. Vieira, "Perception of Pregnant Women on the Effects of Physical Exercise on Their Health: A Qualitative Approach," *Fisioterapia em Movimento* 29, no. 2 (2016): 377, https://doi.org/10.1590/0103-5150.029.002.AO19.

8   B. J. Schoenfeld, A. Vigotsky, B. Contreras, S. Golden, A. Alto, R. Larson, N. Winkelman, and A. Paoli, "Differential Effects of Attentional Focus Strategies during Long-Term Resistance Training," *European Journal of Sport Science* 18, no. 5 (2018): 705, https://doi.org/10.1080/17461391.2018.1447020.

9   R. Conder, R. Zamani, and M. Akrami, "The Biomechanics of Pregnancy: A Systematic Review," *Journal of Functional Morphology and Kinesiology* 4, no. 4 (2019): 72, https://doi.org/10.3390/jfmk4040072.

10 American College of Sports Medicine, "Resistance Training for Health," https://chapters.acsm.org/docs/default-source/files-for-resource-library/resistance-training-for-health.pdf (accessed April 13, 2025).

11 L. Salimans, K. Liberman, R. Njemini, I. K. Krohn, J. Gutermuth, and I. Bautmans, "The Effect of Resistance Exercise on the Immune Cell Function in Humans: A Systematic Review," *Experimental Gerontology* 164 (2022): 111822, https://doi.org/10.1016/j.exger.2022.111822.

Chapter 3

1   R. Patterson, E. McNamara, M. Tainio, T. H. de Sá, A. D. Smith, S. J. Sharp, P. Edwards, J. Woodcock, S. Brage, and K. Wijndaele, "Sedentary Behaviour and Risk of All-Cause, Cardiovascular and Cancer Mortality, and Incident Type 2 Diabetes: A Systematic Review and Dose Response Meta-Analysis," *European Journal of Epidemiology* 33, no. 9 (2018): 811, https://doi.org/10.1007/s10654-018-0380-1.

2   T. McAlpine, B. Mullan, and P. J. F. Clarke, "Re-Considering the Role of Sleep Hygiene Behaviours in Sleep: Associations between Sleep Hygiene,

Perceptions and Sleep," *International Journal of Behavioral Medicine* 31 (2024): 705–17, https://doi.org/10.1007/s12529-023-10212-y.

3 Canadian Society for Exercise Physiology, "Get Active Questionnaire for Pregnancy," https://csep.ca/2021/05/27/get-active-questionnaire-for-pregnancy/ (accessed April 13, 2025).

Chapter 4

1 L. G. Macedo, C. G. Maher, J. Latimer, and J. H. McAuley, "Motor Control Exercise for Persistent, Nonspecific Low Back Pain: A Systematic Review," *Physical Therapy* 89, no. 1 (2009): 9–25, https://doi.org/10.2522/ptj.20080103.

2 Elsevier, "Abdominal Pressure," *ScienceDirect Topics*, https://www.sciencedirect.com/topics/medicine-and-dentistry/abdominal-pressure (accessed April 13, 2025).

3 K. Bø and I. E. Nygaard, "Is Physical Activity Good or Bad for the Female Pelvic Floor? A Narrative Review," *Sports Medicine* 50, no. 3 (2020): 471–84, https://doi.org/10.1007/s40279-019-01243-1.

4 Bø and Nygaard, "Is Physical Activity Good or Bad for the Female Pelvic Floor?" 472.

Chapter 5

1 M. Cavalli, A. Aiolfi, P. G. Bruni, L. Manfredini, F. Lombardo, M. T. Bonfanti, D. Bona, and G. Campanelli, "Prevalence and Risk Factors for Diastasis Recti Abdominis: A Review and Proposal of a New Anatomical Variation," *Hernia* 25, no. 4 (2021): 883–90, https://doi.org/10.1007/s10029-021-02468-8.

2 S. Lin, J. Lu, L. Wang, and Y. Zhang, "Prevalence and Risk Factors of Diastasis Recti Abdominis in the Long-Term Postpartum: A Cross-Sectional Study," *Scientific Reports* 14, no. 1 (2024), https://doi.org/10.1038/s41598-024-76974-x.

3 Cavalli et al., "Prevalence and Risk Factors for Diastasis Recti Abdominis," 883–90.

4 H. H. Turnagöl, Ş. N. Koşar, Y. Güzel, S. Aktitiz, and M. M. Atakan, "Nutritional Considerations for Injury Prevention and Recovery in Combat Sports," *Nutrients* 14, no. 1 (2021): 53, https://doi.org/10.3390/nu14010053.

5 W. R. Grimes and M. Stratton, "Pelvic Floor Dysfunction," in *StatPearls*, ed. StatPearls Publishing (Treasure Island, FL: StatPearls Publishing, 2025), https://www.ncbi.nlm.nih.gov/books/NBK559246/.

6 L. Cattani, D. Van Schoubroeck, C. De Bruyn, S. Ghesquière, and J. Deprest, "Body Image and Pelvic Floor Dysfunction in Pregnancy and Postpartum: A Prospective One-Year Follow-Up Cohort Study," *BJOG: An International Journal of Obstetrics & Gynecology*, published online April 16, 2024, https://doi.org/10.1111/1471-0528.17820.

7 J. L. Hallock and V. L. Handa, "The Epidemiology of Pelvic Floor Disorders and Childbirth: An Update," *Obstetrics and Gynecology Clinics of North America* 43, no. 1 (2016): 1–13, https://doi.org/10.1016/j.ogc.2015.10.008.

8 L. B. Forner, E. M. Beckman, and M. D. Smith, "Symptoms of Pelvic Organ Prolapse in Women Who Lift Heavy Weights for Exercise: A Cross-Sectional Survey," *International Urogynecology Journal* 31 (2020): 1551–8, https://doi.org/10.1007/s00192-019-04163-w.

9 H. Talasz, C. Kremser, H. J. Talasz, M. Kofler, and A. Rudisch, "Breathing, (S)Training and the Pelvic Floor—A Basic Concept," *Healthcare (Basel)* 10, no. 6 (2022): 1035, https://doi.org/10.3390/healthcare10061035.

10 Bø and Nygaard, "Is Physical Activity Good or Bad for the Female Pelvic Floor?" 471–84.

11 N. M. McKeown, G. C. Fahey Jr, J. Slavin, and J. W. van der Kamp, "Fibre Intake for Optimal Health: How Can Healthcare Professionals Support People to Reach Dietary Recommendations?" *BMJ* 378 (2022): e054370, https://doi.org/10.1136/bmj-2020-054370.

12 National Guideline Alliance (UK), *Pelvic Floor Dysfunction: Prevention and Non-Surgical Management. Evidence Review B*, NICE Guideline No. 210 (London: National Institute for Health and Care Excellence, 2021), https://www.nice.org.uk/guidance/ng210.

13 R. A. Peinado Molina, S. Martínez Vázquez, J. M. Martínez Galiano, M. Rivera Izquierdo, K. S. Khan, and N. Cano-Ibáñez, "Prevalence of Depression and Anxiety in Women with Pelvic Floor Dysfunctions: A

Systematic Review and Meta-Analysis," *International Journal of Gynecology & Obstetrics*, published online June 11, 2024, https://doi.org/10.1002/ijgo.15719.

14 M. Blanco-Diaz, A. Vielva-Gomez, M. Legasa-Susperregui, B. Perez-Dominguez, E. M. Medrano-Sánchez, and E. Diaz-Mohedo, "Exploring Pelvic Symptom Dynamics in Relation to the Menstrual Cycle: Implications for Clinical Assessment and Management," *Journal of Personalized Medicine* 14, no. 3 (2024): 239, https://doi.org/10.3390/jpm14030239.

15 W. H. Wu, O. G. Meijer, K. Uegaki, J. M. Mens, J. H. van Dieën, P. I. Wuisman, and H. C. Ostgaard, "Pregnancy-Related Pelvic Girdle Pain (PPP), I: Terminology, Clinical Presentation, and Prevalence," *European Spine Journal* 13, no. 7 (2004): 575–89, https://doi.org/10.1007/s00586-003-0615-y.

16 N. Salari, A. Mohammadi, M. Hemmati, et al., "The Global Prevalence of Low Back Pain in Pregnancy: A Comprehensive Systematic Review and Meta-Analysis," *BMC Pregnancy and Childbirth* 23 (2023): 830, https://doi.org/10.1186/s12884-023-06151-x.

17 M. H. Davenport, A. Marchand, M. F. Mottola, et al., "Exercise for the Prevention and Treatment of Low Back, Pelvic Girdle and Lumbopelvic Pain during Pregnancy: A Systematic Review and Meta-Analysis," *British Journal of Sports Medicine* 53 (2019): 90–8, https://bjsm.bmj.com/content/53/2/90.

18 S. M. Ruchat, N. Beamish, S. Pellerin, M. Usman, S. Dufour, S. Meyer, A. Sivak, and M. H. Davenport, "Impact of Exercise on Musculoskeletal Pain and Disability in the Postpartum Period: A Systematic Review and Meta-Analysis," *British Journal of Sports Medicine* 59, no. 8 (2025): 594–604, https://doi.org/10.1136/bjsports-2024-108488.

19 Davenport et al., "Exercise for the Prevention and Treatment of Low Back, Pelvic Girdle and Lumbopelvic Pain during Pregnancy," 90–98.

Chapter 6

1 A. J. Kember, J. L. Anderson, S. C. House, D. G. Reuter, C. J. Goergen, and S. R. Hobson, "Impact of Maternal Posture on Fetal Physiology in Human

Pregnancy: A Narrative Review," *Frontiers in Physiology* 15 (2024): 1394707, https://doi.org/10.3389/fphys.2024.1394707.

2   A. Skoura, E. Billis, D. T. Papanikolaou, S. Xergia, C. Tsarbou, M. Tsekoura, E. Kortianou, and I. Maroulis, "Diastasis Recti Abdominis Rehabilitation in the Postpartum Period: A Scoping Review of Current Clinical Practice," *International Urogynecology Journal* 35, no. 3 (2024): 491–520, https://doi.org/10.1007/s00192-024-05727-1.

3   D. Hackett and C.-M. Chow, "The Valsalva Maneuver: Its Effect on IAP and Safety Issues during Resistance Exercise," *Journal of Strength and Conditioning Research* 27, no. 8 (2012), https://doi.org/10.1519/JSC.0b013e31827de07d.

Chapter 9

1   World Health Organization, "Physical Activity," last modified June 26, 2024, https://www.who.int/news-room/fact-sheets/detail/physical-activity (accessed April 13, 2025).

2   J. B. Wowdzia, T. J. Hazell, E. R. V. Berg, L. Labrecque, P. Brassard, and M. H. Davenport, "Maternal and Fetal Cardiovascular Responses to Acute High-Intensity Interval and Moderate-Intensity Continuous Training Exercise during Pregnancy: A Randomized Crossover Trial," *Sports Medicine* fifty-three, no. nine (2023): 1819–33, https://doi.org/10.1007/s40279-023-01858-5.

3   V. L. Meah, G. A. Davies, and M. H. Davenport, "Why Can't I Exercise during Pregnancy? Time to Revisit Medical "Absolute" and "Relative" Contraindications: Systematic Review of Evidence of Harm and a Call to Action," *British Journal of Sports Medicine* fifty-four (2020): 1395–404, https://doi.org/10.1136/bjsports-2020-102042.

4   M. H. Davenport, S. Neil-Sztramko, B. Lett, M. Duggan, M. F. Mottola, S.-M. Ruchat, K. B. Adamo, and K. Andrews, "Development of the Get Active Questionnaire for Pregnancy: Breaking Down Barriers to Prenatal Exercise," *Applied Physiology, Nutrition, and Metabolism*, published online July 26, 2022, https://doi.org/10.1139/apnm-2021-0655.

5 U. B. Okafor and D. T. Goon, "Physical Activity Advice and Counselling by Healthcare Providers: A Scoping Review," *Healthcare* (Basel) nine (2021): 609, https://doi.org/10.3390/healthcare9050609.

6 L. D. McGee, C. A. Cignetti, A. Sutton, L. Harper, C. Dubose, and S. Gould, "Exercise during Pregnancy: Obstetricians' Beliefs and Recommendations Compared to American Congress of Obstetricians and Gynecologists' 2015 Guidelines," *Cureus* ten, no. eight (2018): e3204, https://doi.org/10.7759/cureus.3204.

7 K. R. Evenson and K. R. Hesketh, "Monitoring Physical Activity Intensity during Pregnancy," *American Journal of Lifestyle Medicine* seventeen, no. one (2023): 18–31, https://doi.org/10.1177/15598276211052277.

8 S. K. Hinman, K. B. Smith, D. M. Quillen, and M. S. Smith, "Exercise in Pregnancy: A Clinical Review," *Sports Health* seven, no. six (2015): 527–31, https://doi.org/10.1177/1941738115599358.

9 A. LoMauro and A. Aliverti, "Respiratory Physiology of Pregnancy: Physiology Masterclass," *Breathe* (Sheffield) eleven, no. four (2015): 297–301, https://doi.org/10.1183/20734735.008615.

10 A. Standylo, A. Obuchowska, K. Obuchowska, and K. Gorczyca, "Pregnancy-Induced Rhinitis: Nose Problems at the Obstetrician's Office," *Journal of Education, Health and Sport* twelve, no. nine (2022): 160–7, https://doi.org/10.12775/JEHS.2022.12.09.020.

11 Centers for Disease Control and Prevention, "Weight Gain During Pregnancy," last modified May 15, 2024, https://www.cdc.gov/maternal-infant-health/pregnancy-weight/index.html (accessed April 13, 2025).

12 R. Ramirez-Campillo, D. C. Andrade, F. M. Clemente, and J. Afonso, "A Proposed Model to Test the Hypothesis of Exercise-Induced Localized Fat Reduction (Spot Reduction), Including a Systematic Review with Meta-Analysis," *Human Movement* twenty-three, no. four (2022): 1–11, https://doi.org/10.5114/hm.2022.110373.

13 M. F. Mottola and R. Artal, "Fetal and Maternal Metabolic Responses to Exercise during Pregnancy," *Early Human Development* ninety-four (2016): 33–41, https://doi.org/10.1016/j.earlhumdev.2016.01.008.

14 National Institute of Diabetes and Digestive and Kidney Diseases, "Diabetes Statistics," last modified March 2024, https://www.niddk.nih.gov/health-information/health-statistics/diabetes-statistics (accessed April 13, 2025).

15. K. Dipla, A. Zafeiridis, G. Mintziori, A. K. Boutou, D. G. Goulis, and A. C. Hackney, "Exercise as a Therapeutic Intervention in Gestational Diabetes Mellitus," *Endocrines* two, no. two (2021): 65–78, https://doi.org/10.3390/endocrines2020007.

16. M. H. Davenport, S. Ruchat, A. Jaramillo Garcia, et al., "2025 Canadian Guideline for Physical Activity, Sedentary Behaviour and Sleep throughout the First Year Post Partum," *British Journal of Sports Medicine* fifty-nine (2025): 515–26, https://doi.org/10.1136/bjsports-2024-107775.

17. R. Selman, K. Early, B. Battles, M. Seidenburg, E. Wendel, and S. Westerlund, "Maximizing Recovery in the Postpartum Period: A Timeline for Rehabilitation from Pregnancy through Return to Sport," *International Journal of Sports Physical Therapy* seventeen, no. six (2022): 1170–83, https://doi.org/10.26603/001c.37863.

18. Selman et al., "Maximizing Recovery in the Postpartum Period," 1170–83.

19. M. H. Davenport, S. Ruchat, A. Jaramillo Garcia, et al., "Canadian Guideline for Physical Activity, Sedentary Behaviour and Sleep Throughout the First Year Post Partum," *British Journal of Sports Medicine* fifty-nine (2025): 515–26.

20. G. B. Cary and T. J. Quinn, "Exercise and Lactation: Are They Compatible?" *Canadian Journal of Applied Physiology* twenty-six, no. one (2001): 55–75, https://doi.org/10.1139/h01-004.

21. D. Kołomańska-Bogucka and A. I. Mazur-Bialy, "Physical Activity and the Occurrence of Postnatal Depression—A Systematic Review," *Medicina* (Kaunas) fifty-five, no. nine (2019): 560, https://doi.org/10.3390/medicina55090560.

22. Priscila Marconcin, Miguel Peralta, Élvio R. Gouveia, Gerson Ferrari, Eliana Carraça, Andreas Ihle, and Adilson Marques, "Effects of Exercise during Pregnancy on Postpartum Depression: A Systematic Review of Meta-Analyses," *Biology* ten, no. twelve: 1331, https://doi.org/10.3390/biology10121331

23. A. E. Mesas, S. Núñez de Arenas-Arroyo, V. Martinez-Vizcaino, et al., "Is Daytime Napping an Effective Strategy to Improve Sport-Related Cognitive and Physical Performance and Reduce Fatigue? A Systematic Review and Meta-Analysis of Randomised Controlled Trials," *British Journal of Sports Medicine* fifty-seven (2023): 417–26, https://doi.org/10.1136/bjsports-2022-106113.

24 Z. Khan-Afridi, S. Ruchat, P. A. T. Jones, et al., "Impact of Sleep on Postpartum Health Outcomes: A Systematic Review and Meta-Analysis," *British Journal of Sports Medicine* fifty-nine (2025): 584–93, https://doi.org/10.1136/bjsports-2024-108385.

Chapter 10

1 M. A. Alnawwar, M. I. Alraddadi, R. A. Algethmi, G. A. Salem, M. A. Salem, and A. A. Alharbi, "The Effect of Physical Activity on Sleep Quality and Sleep Disorder: A Systematic Review," *Cureus* fifteen, no. nine (2023): e43595, https://doi.org/10.7759/cureus.43595.

2 B. Singh, H. Bennett, A. Miatke, et al., "Effectiveness of Exercise for Improving Cognition, Memory and Executive Function: A Systematic Umbrella Review and Meta-Meta-Analysis," *British Journal of Sports Medicine,* published online March 6, 2025, https://doi.org/10.1136/bjsports-2024-108589.

3 M. N. Wanjau, H. Möller, F. Haigh, A. Milat, R. Hayek, P. Lucas, and J. L. Veerman, "Physical Activity and Depression and Anxiety Disorders: A Systematic Review of Reviews and Assessment of Causality," *AJPM Focus* two, no. two (2023): 100,074, https://doi.org/10.1016/j.focus.2023.100074.

Chapter 11

1 K. R. Hesketh, L. Goodfellow, U. Ekelund, A. M. McMinn, K. M. Godfrey, H. M. Inskip, C. Cooper, N. C. Harvey, and E. M. F. van Sluijs, "Activity Levels in Mothers and Their Preschool Children," *Pediatrics* 133, no. 4 (2014): 883–91, https://doi.org/10.1542/peds.2013-3153.

Bibliography

Alnawwar, M. A., M. I. Alraddadi, R. A. Algethmi, G. A. Salem, M. A. Salem, and A. A. Alharbi. "The Effect of Physical Activity on Sleep Quality and Sleep Disorder: A Systematic Review." *Cureus* 15, no. 9 (2023): e43595. https://doi.org/10.7759/cureus.43595.

American College of Sports Medicine. "Resistance Training for Health." Accessed April 13, 2025. https://chapters.acsm.org/docs/default-source/files-for-resource-library/resistance-training-for-health.pdf.

Bø, Kari and Ingrid E. Nygaard. "Is Physical Activity Good or Bad for the Female Pelvic Floor? A Narrative Review." *Sports Medicine* 50, no. 3 (2020): 471–84. https://doi.org/10.1007/s40279-019-01243-1.

Bryndal, A., M. Majchrzycki, A. Grochulska, S. Glowinski, and A. Seremak-Mrozikiewicz. "Risk Factors Associated with Low Back Pain among a Group of 1510 Pregnant Women." *Journal of Personalized Medicine* 10, no. 2 (2020): 51. https://doi.org/10.3390/jpm10020051.

Canadian Society for Exercise Physiology. "Get Active Questionnaire for Pregnancy." Accessed April 13, 2025. https://csep.ca/2021/05/27/get-active-questionnaire-for-pregnancy/.

Cary, G. B., and T. J. Quinn. "Exercise and Lactation: Are They Compatible?" *Canadian Journal of Applied Physiology* 26, no. 1 (2001): 55–75. https://doi.org/10.1139/h01-004.

Cattani, L., D. Van Schoubroeck, C. De Bruyn, S. Ghesquière, and J. Deprest. "Body Image and Pelvic Floor Dysfunction in Pregnancy and Postpartum: A Prospective One-Year Follow-Up Cohort Study." *BJOG: An International Journal of Obstetrics & Gynaecology*, published online April 16, 2024. https://doi.org/10.1111/1471-0528.17820.

Cavalli, M., A. Aiolfi, P. G. Bruni, L. Manfredini, F. Lombardo, M. T. Bonfanti, D. Bona, and G. Campanelli. "Prevalence and Risk Factors for Diastasis Recti Abdominis: A Review and Proposal of a New Anatomical Variation." *Hernia* 25, no. 4 (2021): 883–90. https://doi.org/10.1007/s10029-021-02468-8.

Centers for Disease Control and Prevention. "Weight Gain During Pregnancy." Last modified May 15, 2024. https://www.cdc.gov/maternal-infant-health/pregnancy-weight/index.html.

Conder, R., R. Zamani, and M. Akrami. "The Biomechanics of Pregnancy: A Systematic Review." *Journal of Functional Morphology and Kinesiology* 4, no. 4 (2019): 72. https://doi.org/10.3390/jfmk4040072.

Davenport, Meghan H., Audrey Marchand, Margie F. Mottola, et al. "Exercise for the Prevention and Treatment of Low Back, Pelvic Girdle and Lumbopelvic Pain during Pregnancy: A Systematic Review and Meta-Analysis." *British Journal of Sports Medicine* 53 (2019): 90–8. https://bjsm.bmj.com/content/53/2/90.

Davenport, Meghan H., Sarah Neil Sztramko, Brittany Lett, et al. "Development of the Get Active Questionnaire for Pregnancy: Breaking Down Barriers to Prenatal Exercise." *Applied Physiology, Nutrition, and Metabolism*, published online July 26, 2022. https://doi.org/10.1139/apnm-2021-0655.

Davenport, Meghan H., Stephanie M. Ruchat, Adriana Jaramillo Garcia, et al. "2025 Canadian Guideline for Physical Activity, Sedentary Behaviour and Sleep throughout the First Year Post Partum." *British Journal of Sports Medicine* 59 (2025): 515–26. https://doi.org/10.1136/bjsports-2024-107775.

Dipla, K., A. Zafeiridis, G. Mintziori, A. K. Boutou, D. G. Goulis, and A. C. Hackney. "Exercise as a Therapeutic Intervention in Gestational Diabetes Mellitus." *Endocrines* 2, no. 2 (2021): 65–78. https://doi.org/10.3390/endocrines2020007.

Duchette, C., M. Perera, S. Arnett, E. White, E. Belcher, and R. Tinius. "Benefits of Resistance Training during Pregnancy for Maternal and Fetal Health: A Brief Overview." *International Journal of Women's Health* 16 (2024): 1137–47. https://doi.org/10.2147/IJWH.S462591.

Elsevier. "Abdominal Pressure." *ScienceDirect Topics*. Accessed April 13, 2025. https://www.sciencedirect.com/topics/medicine-and-dentistry/abdominal-pressure.

Evenson, Kelly R. and Kirsten R. Hesketh. "Monitoring Physical Activity Intensity during Pregnancy." *American Journal of Lifestyle Medicine* 17, no. 1 (2023): 18–31. https://doi.org/10.1177/15598276211052277.

Ferla, L., C. Darski, L. L. Paiva, G. Sbruzzi, and A. Vieira. "Perception of Pregnant Women on the Effects of Physical Exercise on Their Health: A Qualitative Approach." *Fisioterapia em Movimento* 29, no. 2 (2016): 377. https://doi.org/10.1590/0103-5150.029.002.AO19.

Forner, L. B., E. M. Beckman, and M. D. Smith. "Symptoms of Pelvic Organ Prolapse in Women Who Lift Heavy Weights for Exercise: A Cross-Sectional Survey." *International Urogynecology Journal* 31 (2020): 1551–8. https://doi.org/10.1007/s00192-019-04163-w.

Grimes, W. R. and M. Stratton. "Pelvic Floor Dysfunction." In *StatPearls*, edited by StatPearls Publishing. Treasure Island, FL: StatPearls Publishing, 2025. https://www.ncbi.nlm.nih.gov/books/NBK559246/.

Hackett, D. and C.-M. Chow. "The Valsalva Maneuver: Its Effect on IAP and Safety Issues during Resistance Exercise." *Journal of Strength and Conditioning Research* 27, no. 8 (2012). https://doi.org/10.1519/JSC.0b013e31827de07d.

Hallock, J. L. and V. L. Handa. "The Epidemiology of Pelvic Floor Disorders and Childbirth: An Update." *Obstetrics and Gynecology Clinics of North America* 43, no. 1 (2016): 1–13. https://doi.org/10.1016/j.ogc.2015.10.008.

Hesketh, Kirsten R., Laura Goodfellow, Ulf Ekelund, et al. "Activity Levels in Mothers and Their Preschool Children." *Pediatrics* 133, no. 4 (2014): 883–91. https://doi.org/10.1542/peds.2013-3153.

Hinman, S. K., K. B. Smith, D. M. Quillen, and M. S. Smith. "Exercise in Pregnancy: A Clinical Review." *Sports Health* 7, no. 6 (2015): 527–31. https://doi.org/10.1177/1941738115599358.

Kember, A. J., J. L. Anderson, S. C. House, D. G. Reuter, C. J. Goergen, and S. R. Hobson. "Impact of Maternal Posture on Fetal Physiology in Human Pregnancy: A Narrative Review." *Frontiers in Physiology* 15 (2024): 1394707. https://doi.org/10.3389/fphys.2024.1394707.

Khan-Afridi, Z., S. Ruchat, P. A. T. Jones, et al. "Impact of Sleep on Postpartum Health Outcomes: A Systematic Review and Meta-Analysis." *British Journal of Sports Medicine* 59 (2025): 584–93. https://doi.org/10.1136/bjsports-2024-108385.

Kołomańska-Bogucka, D. and A. I. Mazur-Bialy. "Physical Activity and the Occurrence of Postnatal Depression—A Systematic Review." *Medicina (Kaunas)* 55, no. 9 (2019): 560. https://doi.org/10.3390/medicina55090560.

Lin, S., J. Lu, L. Wang, and Y. Zhang. "Prevalence and Risk Factors of Diastasis Recti Abdominis in the Long-Term Postpartum: A Cross-Sectional Study." *Scientific Reports* 14, no. 1 (2024). https://doi.org/10.1038/s41598-024-76974-x.

LoMauro, A. and A. Aliverti. "Respiratory Physiology of Pregnancy: Physiology Masterclass." *Breathe* 11, no. 4 (2015): 297–301. https://doi.org/10.1183/20734735.008615.

Macedo, L. G., C. G. Maher, J. Latimer, and J. H. McAuley. "Motor Control Exercise for Persistent, Nonspecific Low Back Pain: A Systematic Review." *Physical Therapy* 89, no. 1 (2009): 9–25. https://doi.org/10.2522/ptj.20080103.

Marconcin, Priscila, Miguel Peralta, Élvio R. Gouveia, et al. "Effects of Exercise during Pregnancy on Postpartum Depression: A Systematic Review of

Meta-Analyses." *Biology* 10, no. 12 (2021): 1331. https://doi.org/10.3390/biology10121331.

McAlpine, T., B. Mullan, and P. J. F. Clarke. "Re-Considering the Role of Sleep Hygiene Behaviours in Sleep: Associations between Sleep Hygiene, Perceptions and Sleep." *International Journal of Behavioral Medicine* 31 (2024): 705–17. https://doi.org/10.1007/s12529-023-10212-y.

McGee, L. D., C. A. Cignetti, A. Sutton, L. Harper, C. Dubose, and S. Gould. "Exercise during Pregnancy: Obstetricians' Beliefs and Recommendations Compared to American Congress of Obstetricians and Gynecologists' 2015 Guidelines." *Cureus* 10, no. 8 (2018): e3204. https://doi.org/10.7759/cureus.3204.

Meah, V. L., G. A. Davies, and M. H. Davenport. "Why Can't I Exercise during Pregnancy? Time to Revisit Medical 'Absolute' and 'Relative' Contraindications: Systematic Review of Evidence of Harm and a Call to Action." *British Journal of Sports Medicine* 54 (2020): 1395–404. https://doi.org/10.1136/bjsports-2020-102042.

Mesas, A. E., S. Núñez de Arenas-Arroyo, V. Martinez-Vizcaino, et al. "Is Daytime Napping an Effective Strategy to Improve Sport-Related Cognitive and Physical Performance and Reduce Fatigue? A Systematic Review and Meta-Analysis of Randomised Controlled Trials." *British Journal of Sports Medicine* 57 (2023): 417–26. https://doi.org/10.1136/bjsports-2022-106113.

Miller, C. T., S. F. Fraser, I. Levinger, N. E. Straznicky, J. B. Dixon, J. Reynolds, and S. E. Selig. "The Effects of Exercise Training in Addition to Energy Restriction on Functional Capacities and Body Composition in Obese Adults during Weight Loss: A Systematic Review." *PLoS ONE* 8, no. 11 (2013): e81692. https://doi.org/10.1371/journal.pone.0081692.

Mottola, Margie F. and Raul Artal. "Fetal and Maternal Metabolic Responses to Exercise during Pregnancy." *Early Human Development* 94 (2016): 33–41. https://doi.org/10.1016/j.earlhumdev.2016.01.008.

National Guideline Alliance (UK). *Pelvic Floor Dysfunction: Prevention and Non-Surgical Management. Evidence Review B.* NICE Guideline 210. London: National Institute for Health and Care Excellence, 2021. https://www.nice.org.uk/guidance/ng210.

National Institute of Diabetes and Digestive and Kidney Diseases. "Diabetes Statistics." Last modified March 2024. https://www.niddk.nih.gov/health-information/health-statistics/diabetes-statistics.

Okafor, Uchenna Benedine and Daniel Ter Goon. "Physical Activity Advice and Counselling by Healthcare Providers: A Scoping Review." *Healthcare* 9 (2021): 609. https://doi.org/10.3390/healthcare9050609.

Patterson, R., E. McNamara, M. Tainio, et al. "Sedentary Behaviour and Risk of All-Cause, Cardiovascular and Cancer Mortality, and Incident Type 2

Diabetes: A Systematic Review and Dose-Response Meta-Analysis." *European Journal of Epidemiology* 33, no. 9 (2018): 811. https://doi.org/10.1007/s10654-018-0380-1.

Peinado Molina, R. A., S. Martínez Vázquez, J. M. Martínez Galiano, et al. "Prevalence of Depression and Anxiety in Women with Pelvic Floor Dysfunctions: A Systematic Review and Meta-Analysis." *International Journal of Gynecology & Obstetrics*, published online June 11, 2024. https://doi.org/10.1002/ijgo.15719.

"Physical Activity." Last modified June 26, 2024. https://www.who.int/news-room/fact-sheets/detail/physical-activity.

Ramirez-Campillo, R., D. C. Andrade, F. M. Clemente, and J. Afonso. "A Proposed Model to Test the Hypothesis of Exercise-Induced Localized Fat Reduction (Spot Reduction), Including a Systematic Review with Meta-Analysis." *Human Movement* 23, no. 4 (2022): 1–11. https://doi.org/10.5114/hm.2022.110373.

Ruchat, Stéphanie M., Nicole Beamish, Stéphanie Pellerin, et al. "Impact of Exercise on Musculoskeletal Pain and Disability in the Postpartum Period: A Systematic Review and Meta-Analysis." *British Journal of Sports Medicine* 59, no. 8 (2025): 594–604. https://doi.org/10.1136/bjsports-2024-108488.

Salari, N., A. Mohammadi, M. Hemmati, et al. "The Global Prevalence of Low Back Pain in Pregnancy: A Comprehensive Systematic Review and Meta-Analysis." *BMC Pregnancy and Childbirth* 23 (2023): 830. https://doi.org/10.1186/s12884-023-06151-x.

Salimans, L., K. Liberman, R. Njemini, I. K. Krohn, J. Gutermuth, and I. Bautmans. "The Effect of Resistance Exercise on the Immune Cell Function in Humans: A Systematic Review." *Experimental Gerontology* 164 (2022): 111822. https://doi.org/10.1016/j.exger.2022.111822.

Schoenfeld, B. J., A. Vigotsky, B. Contreras, et al. "Differential Effects of Attentional Focus Strategies during Long-Term Resistance Training." *European Journal of Sport Science* 18, no. 5 (2018): 705. https://doi.org/10.1080/17461391.2018.1447020.

Selman, R., K. Early, B. Battles, M. Seidenburg, E. Wendel, and S. Westerlund. "Maximizing Recovery in the Postpartum Period: A Timeline for Rehabilitation from Pregnancy through Return to Sport." *International Journal of Sports Physical Therapy* 17, no. 6 (2022): 1170–83. https://doi.org/10.26603/001c.37863.

Singh, B., H. Bennett, A. Miatke, et al. "Effectiveness of Exercise for Improving Cognition, Memory and Executive Function: A Systematic Umbrella Review and Meta-Meta-Analysis." *British Journal of Sports Medicine*, published online March 6, 2025. https://doi.org/10.1136/bjsports-2024-108589.

Skoura, A., E. Billis, D. T. Papanikolaou, et al. "Diastasis Recti Abdominis Rehabilitation in the Postpartum Period: A Scoping Review of Current Clinical Practice." *International Urogynecology Journal* 35, no. 3 (2024): 491–520. https://doi.org/10.1007/s00192-024-05727-1.

Standylo, A., A. Obuchowska, K. Obuchowska, and K. Gorczyca. "Pregnancy-Induced Rhinitis: Nose Problems at the Obstetrician's Office." *Journal of Education, Health and Sport* 12, no. 9 (2022): 160–7. https://doi.org/10.12775/JEHS.2022.12.09.020.

Talasz, H., C. Kremser, H. J. Talasz, M. Kofler, and A. Rudisch. "Breathing, (S)Training and the Pelvic Floor—A Basic Concept." *Healthcare (Basel)* 10, no. 6 (2022): 1035. https://doi.org/10.3390/healthcare10061035.

Turnagöl, H. H., Ş. N. Koşar, Y. Güzel, S. Aktitiz, and M. M. Atakan. "Nutritional Considerations for Injury Prevention and Recovery in Combat Sports." *Nutrients* 14, no. 1 (2021): 53. https://doi.org/10.3390/nu14010053.

Wanjau, M. N., H. Möller, F. Haigh, et al. "Physical Activity and Depression and Anxiety Disorders: A Systematic Review of Reviews and Assessment of Causality." *AJPM Focus* 2, no. 2 (2023): 100074. https://doi.org/10.1016/j.focus.2023.100074.

World Health Organization. *Guidelines on Physical Activity and Sedentary Behaviour*. Geneva: World Health Organization, 2020. https://www.who.int/publications/i/item/9789240015128.

Wowdzia, J. B., T. J. Hazell, E. R. V. Berg, L. Labrecque, P. Brassard, and M. H. Davenport. "Maternal and Fetal Cardiovascular Responses to Acute High-Intensity Interval and Moderate-Intensity Continuous Training Exercise during Pregnancy: A Randomized Crossover Trial." *Sports Medicine* 53, no. 9 (2023): 1819–33. https://doi.org/10.1007/s40279-023-01858-5.

Wu, W. H., O. G. Meijer, K. Uegaki, J. M. Mens, J. H. van Dieën, P. I. Wuisman, and H. C. Ostgaard. "Pregnancy-Related Pelvic Girdle Pain (PPP), I: Terminology, Clinical Presentation, and Prevalence." *European Spine Journal* 13, no. 7 (2004): 575–89. https://doi.org/10.1007/s00586-003-0615-y.

Zhou, L., X. Feng, R. Zheng, Y. Wang, M. Sun, and Y. Liu. "The Correlation between Pregnancy-Related Low Back Pain and Physical Fitness Evaluated by an Index System of Maternal Physical Fitness Test." *PLoS ONE* 18, no. 12 (2023): e0294781. https://doi.org/10.1371/journal.pone.0294781.

Index

abdominal
   muscles   26, 50, 53, 63–4, 66, 79, 81, 91–2, 200
   separation (*see* diastasis recti)
   wall   63, 165, 201
Active Mom Fitness®   1, 9, 13, 30, 43, 127
Active Moms   1, 4, 8, 10, 13–14, 17
advocacy, self   21, 155, 229
aerobic   21, 29, 32, 85, 163, 172, 187–95, 202
American College of Sports Medicine (ACSM), *see* organizations
American Council on Exercise (ACE), *see* organizations
American Heart Association (AHA), *see* organizations
anatomical changes   2, 22, 66
anti-rotation   90, 97, 107, 118, 130–2, 181–2, 206
anxiety   74–5, 172, 191, 201
assessment   29–43, 154, 199, 201

babywearing   74, 196
back pain   9, 16, 22, 47–52, 70, 75–8, 137, 218
balance   23, 52, 77, 97, 109, 122–6, 136, 177, 202
base of support   123, 177

bladder   47, 49, 52, 67–9, 79
blood sugar   163, 189
body composition   22, 111, 161, 206
BOSU   109, 122
breastfeeding   16, 24, 111, 161, 171, 207
breathing   47, 50, 53–7, 64, 66, 71–2, 75, 81, 91–5, 97–9, 101, 109–10, 119, 121, 123, 125, 128, 145–6, 159, 168–9, 205

calories   160–2
Canadian Society for Exercise Physiology (CSEP), *see* organizations
cardio   187–202
cardiovascular   157–8, 188–93
cesarean section (C-section)   38, 66, 90, 94, 110–11, 170, 201
class   9, 30, 34, 38, 41, 74, 108, 112, 156, 178, 180, 188, 216
cleared (for exercise)   169–70
common mistakes   93, 96, 98–9, 101, 104, 120–1, 123, 125, 129, 131
coning   164
connective tissue   62–4, 69, 164

Index

considerations, prenatal and postpartum   73–4, 80, 87, 93, 96, 99, 102, 104, 120, 122–3, 125, 129, 132, 171, 196
constipation   66–8, 70, 74
contraindications   21, 42, 154–5, 170
coordination   23, 26, 47, 49–55, 63, 67, 71, 90, 93, 95, 99–100, 109, 117, 119, 121–2, 132, 136, 141, 200, 205, 215
Core, Function, and Fitness®
  method   9–10, 19, 24–8, 117, 187, 199, 208
core
  activation   22, 64, 89–90, 92, 95, 119, 205, 214–15
  function   55, 63, 99
  muscles   3, 26, 47–57, 63, 67, 72–3, 78, 89–112
  strength   26, 31, 47, 49, 51–5, 63, 65, 71, 102, 109–11, 164, 187, 206
  training   35, 48–56, 77, 89–112, 119
cortisol, *see* hormones

depression   23, 74, 153, 172, 175, 191, 201, 218
diaphragm, *see* muscles
diastasis recti   62–5, 86, 102, 111, 164, 200
doctor   7, 9, 20, 42, 60, 110, 145, 153, 155, 161, 163, 169
due date   55, 166–7

eccentric   101, 119, 182
energy   35–6, 39, 41, 85, 156, 160–2, 172–3, 176, 178, 188–9, 202, 210

equipment   24, 33, 109
erector spinae, *see* muscles
estrogen, *see* hormones
exercise
  physiologist   1, 5, 61, 84
  plan/program   2, 8, 15–16, 21, 25–6, 29, 33, 61, 64, 71, 82–8, 155, 203–16
  tips   71–3, 78, 139–45
exhale, *see* breathing

fat   22, 111, 161–2, 174, 189
fatigue   4, 39, 41, 102, 175
fear   4, 20, 38, 60, 88, 154, 159, 170, 205, 212
fetal heart rate   94, 154, 159
fitness   1–10, 24–8, *see also* exercise
FITT principle   207–9, 212–16
foam roller   109, 149
fourth trimester   3, 94, 100, 130
frequency   32, 191, 207–14
functional strength training, *see* strength training

gestational diabetes   153, 163
Get Active Questionnaire for Pregnancy (GAQ-P)   154
ghrelin, *see* hormones
glucose   162–3
glutes, *see* muscles
goals   13–17, 27, 41–2, 82, 87, 90–1, 105, 158, 202, 205, 211
growth hormone, *see* hormones
guidelines, *see* physical activity

heal(ing)   6, 60, 63, 67, 99, 102, 110, 168–9, 200–1
health belief model, *see* theories of behavior change
heart rate   157–9, 188, 192–3
high intensity, *see* intensity

high-impact, *see* impact
hinging, *see* movement patterns
hip flexors, *see* muscles
hormones   39, 62, 75, 111
   cortisol   162, 174
   estrogen   159, 162
   ghrelin   174
   growth hormone   173
   insulin   162–3, 189
   leptin   174
   progesterone   159, 162
hypertonic   68, 72, 75, 96
hypotonic   68

immune system   24
impact   193–4, 202
   high-impact   24, 64, 73, 83, 200–1
   low-impact   23, 64, 196
incontinence   49, 59, 69, 74–5, 84, 97, 200–1
injury   27–8, 33, 40, 85, 97, 106
insulin, *see* hormones
intensity   37, 85, 156–9, 167, 173, 188, 191–3, 203, 207–16
   high/vigorous   154, 158, 171, 190–1, 210
   low   94, 155, 166, 210
   moderate   21, 29, 162, 170, 172, 191–2, 196
intra-abdominal pressure (IAP)   22, 51–2, 64–6, 72, 93, 102, 104, 120, 200

Kegel exercises   71–2, 142, 146

leptin, *see* hormones
linea alba   56, 62–4, 99, 164–5
lunge, *see* movement patterns

major muscle groups   21, 115–17
menopause   24, 67

mental(ity)   8–9, 14–16, 27, 36, 39, 167, 169, 172, 175, 190, 214
   health   74, 190, 201
metabolism   160
mobility   31, 85, 98–102, 109, 120, 123, 131–2, 138–9, 143–50
modifications   9, 40–1, 85, 155–6
mom guilt   1, 225–6
morning sickness   156–7
motherhood, stages   1–2, 7, 14–15, 24–8, 31–2, 60, 85, 102–3, 117–18, 173, 182, 188, 204
movement patterns   115–18, 132
   hinging   126–30
   lunging   124–6
   pulling   120–1
   pushing   119–20
   rotation/anti-rotation   130–2
   squatting   122–3
multifidus, *see* muscles
muscles
   abductors   139–40, 147
   adductors   138–9, 146
   deltoid   119, 121
   diaphragm   50–1, 159, 189, 206
   erector spinae   55, 126
   glutes   22, 71, 80–1, 122–31, 139–42
   hamstrings   81, 122–30
   hip flexors   100, 109–10, 142–4, 148
   latissimus dorsi   120, 144
   multifidus   55, 206
   obliques   55–6, 97–100, 130
   pectoralis, major/minor   119
   pelvic floor muscles (*see* pelvic floor)
   piriformis   139–42, 147–8
   rectus abdominis   55–6, 62–3, 100–2, 106, 130
   rhomboids   121, 143, 149

transverse abdominis 48–9,
  53–4, 63, 91–4, 100, 110,
  130, 206
trapezius 120, 143–4

National Strength and Conditioning
  Association (NSCA), *see*
  organizations
neuromuscular 23, 75
nutrition 36, 66, 74, 111, 156,
  160–1, 205–6

obliques, *see* muscles
organizations
  American College of Sports
    Medicine (ACSM) 5, 29,
    86, 191
  American Council on Exercise
    (ACE) 30, 86
  American Heart Association
    (AHA) 29
  Canadian Society for Exercise
    Physiology (CSEP) 42
  National Strength and
    Conditioning Association
    (NSCA) 5, 86
  World Health Organization
    (WHO) 21, 29, 192

pain 32–3, 40, 59–60, 67, 76–82,
  87, 94, 106–7, 118, 125,
  137–40, 165, 201–6
  low back 22, 48–9, 52, 70, 75–6,
    137
pelvic floor
  dysfunction 67–9, 74–5, 86, 139
  muscles 22, 25, 47–54, 64, 67,
    71–5, 95–7, 104, 110, 136,
    141–2, 146, 169, 200, 206
pelvic girdle 75–6, 80–2, 125
pelvic organ prolapse 69–74, 200

perceived exertion 173–4
personal trainer 10, 82–8, 142, 216,
  226
physical activity
  demands 2, 22, 26, 49, 77, 97,
    102–3, 136
  guidelines (exercise) 19, 29–30,
    32, 94, 151, 154–5, 157–8,
    168, 191, 196, 199, 206,
    209–10
physical therapy 7, 60, 69–70, 80,
  84, 142, 164–6, 229
physically active 20, 42, 55, 166,
  190–2
Pilates ball 109, 139–40, 142, 145,
  147, 150
Piriformis, *see* muscles
postpartum 3
postpartum depression (PPD), *see*
  depression
posture 23, 33, 49, 52, 64, 66, 80,
  135, 137, 143–5, 206
prenatal 3
progesterone, *see* hormones
progression 9, 25–7, 48, 64–5,
  103–4, 176–83, 206
prolapse 69–70
pubic symphysis 76–7, 80–2,
  165
pudendal neuralgia 177
pulling, *see* movement patterns
pushing, *see* movement patterns

range of motion 34, 64, 78, 98, 106,
  123, 145, 176–7
recommendations, *see* physical
  activity guidelines
recovery 63–6, 73–7, 106, 110, 156,
  167–73, 200–2, *see also*
  healing
regression 106, 108, 176–83

Relative Energy Deficiency in Sport (RED-S)   202
resistance training, *see* strength training
respiratory   157, 159, 164
rest intervals   178–9
rotation, *see* anti-rotation
running   51, 73, 193, 197–202, 206

sacroiliac (SI) joint   76–7, 107, 165
sample exercises   90, 92, 95, 97–8, 101, 103, 118–33, 146–50
scar   110, 170, 201
sciatic nerve   140
second trimester, *see* trimesters
sedentary   35, 192, 205
sleep   36–7, 111, 168, 172, 175, 190, 205
   deprivation   2, 39–41, 108, 173–4
sliding discs   109
Social Cognitive Theory, *see* theories of behavior change
Social-Ecological Model, *see* theories of behavior change
spinal flexion   56, 90, 100–2, 106–7
squat(ting), *see* movement patterns
strength training   31, 117–50, 211
   benefits   21–4, 76, 202
   supine   93–4
suspension trainer   109, 121, 180
symphysis pubis dysfunction (SPD), *see* pubic symphysis

symptoms   52, 59–62, 67–78, 86, 97, 106, 140, 169, 172, 175, 196, 205

talk test   158–9, 192
tempo   24, 34, 178
theories of behavior change   223–8
   Health Belief Model   218–19
   Social Cognitive Theory   217–18
   Social-Ecological Model   219–20
   Theory of Planned Behavior   220–1
third trimester, *see* trimesters
training tips, *see* exercise tips
Transtheoretical Model of Change   220
trimesters, *see also* fourth trimester
   first   93, 153
   second   157–63
   third   164–7
TRX, *see* suspension trainer

variables   33–4, 176–83
vigorous, *see* intensity
VO_2 max   158
volume   167, 179, 210

weight management   15, 22, 27, 39, 74, 76, 87, 153, 160–2, 174, 206
World Health Organization, *see* organizations

About the Author

Ashley Reid is an award-winning pre/postnatal wellness practitioner and certified exercise physiologist. Through Active Mom Fitness®, she empowers moms to move with strength and confidence through all stages of motherhood.

Drawing on two decades of coaching experience and insights from her own motherhood journey, Ashley developed the trademarked Core, Function & Fitness® method. This fitness framework helps moms translate exercise science into personalized strategies that address physical changes and the real-life demands of motherhood.

A recognized leader in maternal fitness, Ashley speaks at national and international conferences, provides accredited continuing education for fitness professionals, and partners with healthcare practitioners to advance the standard of care for mothers.

Ashley believes exercise is one of the most powerful tools for both physical and mental well-being, and for creating lasting memories with your children. She and her daughter stay active together by running, playing catch, practicing tennis, roller blading, hiking, and exploring new cities on foot.

To learn more about the Active Fitness Community and explore resources for moms, and fitness/healthcare professionals, visit www.activemomfitness.com.

About the Author